I0568611

BOOK ONE

THE

Word

ON

Weight LOSS

Faith-based weight loss tips, tools & strategies

CATHY MORENZIE

GUIDING
LIGHT
PRESS

Published: April 2022

ISBN: (print) 978-1-990078-10-1

(digital) 978-1-990078-11-8

Published by Guiding Light Publishing

46 Bell St, Barrie, ON, Canada, L4N 0H9

Note: The information in this book is for educational purposes only and is not recommended as a means of diagnosing or treating illness. All situations concerning physical or mental health should be supervised by a health professional knowledgeable in treating that particular condition. Neither the author nor anyone affiliated with Healthy by Design dispenses medical advice, nor do they prescribe any remedies or assume any responsibility for anyone who chooses to treat themselves.

Cover and author photo by: martinbrownphotography.com

Cover design by: kimmontefortedesign.com

Interior Design by: Davor Dramikanin

Table of Contents

Chapter Five

The Word on Weight Loss

Also by Cathy Morenzie

The Breakthrough Method
Your Guided Path to Weight Loss God's Way

Spirit-Filled & Sugar-Free:
30 Day Sugar Detox Devotional and Weight Loss Plan

Weight Loss, God's Way:
The Proven 21-Day Weight Loss Devotional Bible Study

Weight Loss, God's Way:
Low-Carb Cookbook and 21-Day Meal Plan

Pray Powerfully, Lose Weight:
21 Days of Short Prayers, Declarations, Scriptures and
Quotes for a Healthy Body, Spirit and Soul

Love God, Lose Weight:
Freedom from Emotional Eating, Overeating and Self-
Sabotage by Accepting God's Love

Get Active, God's Way:
Weight Loss Devotional and Workout Challenge

Healthy Eating, God's Way:
Weight Loss Devotional and Challenge

A Note From The Author

Dear Reader,

Thank you for joining me on this journey to better health through "The WORD on Weight Loss." My heart is to help you not only shed pounds but to grow stronger in your faith, renew your mind, and heal emotionally. This book is designed to provide you with the tools and encouragement you need to succeed in every aspect of your weight loss journey.

By embracing the biblical principles and practical tips shared in these pages, you'll discover how to align your health goals with God's purpose for your life, finding strength in His Word. You will renew your mind to overcome obstacles and develop a positive, can-do attitude. Additionally, you will address the root causes of emotional eating and learn to manage your feelings in a healthy way.

As a token of my appreciation for your commitment, I'm thrilled to offer you an exclusive bonus. Visit weightlossgodswaybonus. com to access:

- Weekly Insights; Exclusive Videos; Special Offers; 70 Simple and Powerful Tips You Can Start Immediately to Lose Weight and much more.

This bonus content is my way of saying thank you for investing in your health and well-being through this book. I pray it will be a valuable resource on your journey.

Remember, you are not alone. Together, with God's guidance, we can achieve the healthy, vibrant life He has planned for us.

Blessings,

Cathy Morenzie

Foreword

When I was asked if I would be willing to help produce this book, a compilation of the very best and most popular of Cathy Morenzie's blog posts from the last decade, I immediately jumped at the chance. Sure it meant reading through hundreds of blog posts to curate the select few that would make it into these pages, but having read some of Cathy's books (from her popular and award-winning Healthy by Design series of weight loss devotionals) I was more than happy to learn all I could from her and, in turn, help you to do the same.

First and foremost, the goal of this book is to help women get healthy, both inside and out. The importance of spiritual and emotional health is clear to many of us. But when it comes to our physical health, sometimes we don't see this as important and worth our time and effort because we assume it is much lower on the totem pole than overall spirituality. We may even think it shouldn't be something a godly woman concerns herself with, so taking time to exercise and eat nutritious food doesn't make it anywhere near our to-do list.

While we won't get into this issue right now, the importance of taking care of our vessels will be addressed in this book. In fact, the first section of *The Word on Weight Loss* will address the spiritual reasons for why our own personal health should be a priority for each woman who seeks to live a godly and productive life.

First off, let's see how Jesus sees us, each one of us, no exceptions.

Hebrews 12:1–2 NRSV: Therefore, since we are surrounded by so great a cloud of witnesses, let us also lay aside every weight and the sin that clings so closely, and let us run with perseverance the race that is set before us, looking to Jesus the pioneer and perfecter of our faith who for the sake of the joy that was set before him endured the cross, disregarding its shame, and has taken his seat at the right hand of the throne of God.

Isaiah 53:5 NRSV: But he was wounded for our transgressions, crushed for our iniquities; upon him was the punishment that made him whole, and by his bruises we are healed.

What are some of the takeaways?

1. We are a joy to Jesus. Whatever weaknesses or failures we've experienced, He paid it all so we can be free from being controlled by any and every sin.

    Have you ever encountered someone willing to do the right thing or help you in some way? How did that make you feel?

    This weekend, my daughter is coming home from college to visit. Since we all tend to use her room for various things while she is away, it can become cluttered, but her younger brother uses it the most. Today I told him I would be cleaning up her room and if he wanted to do it together, that would be great.

    His response was, "I am planning on cleaning her room up and also her bathroom." He did this the last time she visited also, but I'd forgotten. It was such a relief to have him in my corner, helping me tidy the house, because I was cleaning the kitchen and other rooms. It made my heart glad and made me feel joyful, knowing my son had not only my back, but his sister's as well.

When we, as children of God, want to help God out by becoming our best for Him and providing an example that others can look to as well, I bet it makes His heart glad also.

2. We can make needed changes; we simply must be willing. He took the pain through His stripes and bruises, and healed us.

Romans 8:11 NRSV: If the Spirit of Him who raised Jesus from the dead dwells in you...

We have the same Spirit and power dwelling in us that raised Jesus Himself from the grave and from the dead. We simply need to plug into that power. The hard work has been done. We must depend upon and rest in His power and not in our own earthly lack of power and self-control.

What we will not be doing in this book is comparing ourselves to others, especially images of women that have been photo-shopped. It's not about looking the best, it is about looking *our* best and doing the best with our own temples, not someone else's.

Here are more scriptures to consider, in case there is even a hint of the spirit of our brother, Doubting Thomas, in anyone reading this.

1 Corinthians 6:19-20 NRSV
Or do you not know that your body is a temple of the Holy Spirit within you, which you have from God, and that you are not your own? For you were bought with a price; therefore, glorify God in your body.

1 Corinthians 6:12 ESV
"All things are lawful for me," but not all things are helpful.
"All things are lawful for me," but I will not be enslaved by
anything.

3 John 1:2 NIV
Dear friend, I pray that you may enjoy good health and
that all may go well with you, even as your soul is getting
along well.

Proverbs 31:17 NRSV
She girds herself with strength and makes her
arms strong.

Proverbs 23:2 ESV
And put a knife to your throat if you are given to appetite.

Galatians 5.22–23 ESV
But the fruit of the Spirit is love, joy, peace, patience,
kindness, goodness, faithfulness, gentleness, self-control;
against such things there is no law.

Proverbs 25:16 NLT
Do you like honey? Don't eat too much, or it will make
you sick!

These scriptures all show us the connection between our spiritual life and our physical bodies. The first thing a lost soul or younger disciple sees is our physical body. Yes, they will know we are Christians by our love, but they will know how devoted we are to following **everything** the Lord commands by whether or not we have taken the time and effort to do the best we can with the temple He has given us. And to take care of that temple.

Many of us want our lives to be as close to the worthy woman in Proverbs 31 as we possibly can. Well, she is described in verse 17 as having arms girded with strength. She needs to be strong for her tasks because these are the physical verbs used to describe her: does, seeks, works, brings, rises, plants, dresses, makes, puts, reaches, supplies, laughs, opens, teaches, looks, does not **eat** the bread of idleness. There are other words used to describe her, but only three have to do with anything mental as opposed to physical: perceives, considers, and doesn't fear.

Perhaps we can be women who consider God's view on our physical health, perceive that this is also part of God's plan for each one of our lives, and we will not give in to fear of any kind when it comes to doing what we are able to do to improve our health.

Whatever way you want to look at the Proverbs 31 woman, there is an awful lot of doing; tasks requiring physical effort to complete. This woman was not lazy. She was hard-working, which means she had to consume the foods needed to give her the stamina required, and she had to take care of herself and make that a priority in order to meet the needs of her husband, children, and those in her circle of influence. And she **was** a woman of influence, qualified to teach others. She aspired to excellence and true worship. A worship that was fulfilled by every aspect of her life, not just the ones that were easy to lay on the altar.

So, before we proceed, let's go ahead and ask ourselves some tough questions:

1. Are you really open to hearing what God has to say about the importance of doing what you can to obtain physical health?

2. Do you have the faith needed to move forward and begin making your physical health a priority in your life? If not, do you want the faith to change?

3. Can you identify anything that has been holding you back from taking personal responsibility for your health and well-being?

4. Do you see that while no food in and of itself is wrong to consume, that being addicted to food, or sugar, when it basically amounts to gluttony, is an ungodly trait and must be repented of?

Even if you couldn't answer "yes" right now to any of the questions above, if you are willing to read further and learn more from someone who is a leading Christian weight loss coach, and to give her suggestions a try, I'm sure you'll begin to see how God loves our whole self and we can show our love of God by caring for that which He's given us.

Next, we will take a deeper look at seeing your health through God's perspective.

Blessings!

Melody Delgado

Preface

Is there really a need for a faith-based or Christian-based program? After all, what makes Christian weight loss any different from anyone else's weight loss?

I've gotta admit that I just cringed as I googled 'Christian Weight Loss Programs.' Yikes, at the top of the list was some weight loss guru telling you that you're fat and that he had the biblical secret to help you lose weight.

Reading the claims on his site really challenged me to examine what service I offer.

I never want to be accused of just slapping a Christian sticker on a weight loss program. My goal is to deliver quality content 100% of the time while being sensitive to the role that the Holy Spirit plays in the lives of Christians. This includes their weight loss.

I recognized the need for offering faith-based weight loss programs in my own life after being involved in the health and wellness industry for almost 25 years.

I'm always surprised when I talk to someone who I would consider a 'spiritual giant' and realize that they have never connected their faith with their health.

My desire is to truly see God as all-powerful, which means that I can rely on Him to help me with my relationships, my finances, and *weight loss challenges*. I want Him to be God of all.

Christian or faith-based weight loss programs do not mean to just pray and the fat will melt away; it does not mean to eat only the foods that the Bible says to eat; nor does it mean that you are a sinner because you're fat. It especially does not mean that Christians have discovered the secret to weight loss (in fact, if you look in our churches, it seems quite the contrary).

To be part of a faith-based weight loss program means:

1. Your motivation to lose weight shifts from a self-focused perspective to an act of worship to God as you understand that your body is His temple.

2. That you really believe that God wants you well and healthy, and you believe that He will help you on your journey if you allow Him.

3. You will ask and trust God to strengthen your willpower, self-discipline, and motivation instead of chasing the next weight loss fad.

4. You will no longer waste hundreds if not thousands of dollars on weight loss gimmicks, because God's plan for health and abundance is simple (and inexpensive).

5. You will be part of a supportive team of like-minded people who also believe in the power of prayer and support.

6. You are not focused on quick fixes and see weight loss as a journey to teach you some valuable lessons about life and God.

7. You will no longer feel the need to hide in shame but begin to understand universal principles such as accountability, reciprocity, and intention.

8. Your faith is strengthened as you submit one of the most intimate parts of your life to your Creator.

9. You will learn what the Bible says about your challenges and issues and how to overcome them.

10. You will get RESULTS. Why? Because when God is your strength, you cannot fail.

If you've been skeptical about faith-based books or programs of any kind, then I encourage you to do your homework before you buy into them. Make sure you will be learning about the Word of God while learning all about healthy eating, exercise, and behavior modification. Praying on its own will not get you results.

***

We may not even be aware of how we use Scripture to minimize the benefits of living a healthy, active lifestyle. It's a shame, because it's when we're healthy, energized, confident, and feeling great that the light of Christ shines even brighter for others to see. It's not vain or in vain to make focusing on your body a priority. In fact, if we don't make time to get healthy, we'll be forced to make time for sickness and disease, and that will take a lot more time and effort in the long run, never mind how much it will limit us in our ability to fully serve in all the ways God wants us to.

We can be extremely short-sighted and forget about the long run of trying to live a long and healthy life so we can do more for God for many more years. We worry—yes, worry—about minutiae and minor details. And even some of us who lead—to our shame!—place this faulty, short-term priority mindset upon other women and transfer the pressure to perform and get quick results onto those we lead. We want results now! We want and need things to happen now!

Says who? God? He calls us to submit to His timing and His plans and goals, and not the other way around. We were made to serve Him and not the other way around, either. We are to seek His guidance and be led by the Spirit. Our lack of really, really understanding this is shown and revealed by our prayers. Do we pray, "Your will be done," or do we rattle off a list of things we want and then get upset when God says "no" or "not yet" or even, "Actually, I want you doing something else entirely."

It's so easy to focus on immediate gratification or immediate results, but this short-sighted thinking undermines our ability to succeed at long term success. In the moment, urgent matters seem so important; always dealing with the urgent keeps us reactive and never frees up time to focus on what really matters. Not every urgent matter should be a priority!

Do you place the priority on service, at the sacrifice of your health? Do you confuse self-care with vanity?

There are two scriptures that can lead us into believing that we should not focus on our physical bodies:

> *"For the Lord sees not as man sees: man looks on the*
> *outward appearance, but the Lord looks on the heart."*
> (1 Samuel 16:7 ESV)

and

> *"For physical training is of some value, but godliness has*
> *value for all things, holding promise for both the present life*
> *and the life to come."* (1 Tim 4:8)

It's true that both of these scriptures place a higher value on our inner man; our heart; our soul. But know that God also cares about our 'outer man', which is how the Bible refers to our bodies. And if we read the second verse carefully, it does say that physical training has value. It does not say what some of us think it says that physical training is unimportant and worthless.

Based on these two scriptures, we can be led to think that God does not care if we're overweight. But I think if we dig deeper, we can see that this is in fact not the case.

Let's look at some of the things that we know for sure that God cares about:

1. **God cares about whatever keeps us from fulfilling our purpose and destiny.** Ephesians 2:10 tells us that, *"We are His workmanship, created in Christ Jesus for good works, which God prepared beforehand that we should walk in them."* (ESV) First, we are His workmanship. How amazing is that? Secondly, He created us for good works, yet we all know people who are so bound by their weight, and they are so unhappy, they physically and emotionally are unable to walk in their anointing because their weight physically stops them. Maybe you're that person. Be encouraged by the thought that God has prepared good works for us to do. Use this knowledge as a goal to get healthier. What has God called you to do? Are you able to do it and do it well?

2. **God cares about what we care about.** One of my favorite scriptures is found in 1 Peter 5:7. *"Cast all your anxiety on Him, because He cares for you."* It reminds me that God cares about everything I care about; everything that worries me and causes me anxiety. Being overweight can be all-consuming. It occupies space and time that God wants. If you're overweight and it's causing you stress and anxiety, then know that God cares about this also. He does not want you stressed or anxious and wants you to get the help you need so you are at peace.

3. **God cares about our total health, not just the spiritual aspects.** In 1 Thes. 5:23, the apostle Paul divides human nature into three parts—spirit, soul, and body, and prays to God on behalf of the converts, *"May God himself, the God of peace, sanctify you through and through. May your whole spirit, soul and body be kept blameless at the coming of our Lord Jesus Christ."* Let us also pray to God that all aspects of our human nature be sanctified and strengthened.

4. **God wants us to glorify Him in our body.** Our physical bodies cause us much trouble. Imagine if we did not have physical bodies. Imagine no insecurity issues, jealousy issues, gluttony issues, lust issues, and the list can go on. Yet our Father saw fit to give us physical bodies that would glorify Him. Our responsibility (reasonable service) is to keep it holy by taking care of it. In Romans 12:1, Paul addresses the crowd by stating: *"I beseech you therefore, brethren, by the mercies of God, that ye present your bodies a living sacrifice, holy, acceptable unto God, which is your reasonable service."* (NKJV)

Yes, He Cares

God most certainly cares if we're overweight, but not in the way that we care. Not in a 'you should be a size 8 not 18' sort of way, or in a way that is overly concerned about whether we're the right proportions or if we can fit into a pair of skinny jeans.

His care and love for us extend far beyond anything that we can comprehend. He cares because He knows that being healthy will have an impact on generations to come. He cares because He knows your outer body is a physical manifestation of what's going on inside your mind and spirit, and He wants to free you of the bondage and challenges that come with it. He cares because taking care of our health (like our finances, relationships, family, and careers) are seeds that, when managed well, increase our capacity for impact and prepare us for greater things to come.

***

In his wisdom, in Psalm 139:23-24, David asks God to search his heart and his thoughts and to point out anything that offends Him.

If you've been forever trying to lose weight, learn from David and let this be the starting point for you, too. Take your hands off the steering wheel of your weight loss efforts and ask the Lord to take command and control.

Below the Surface

Ask Him to show you what lies beneath the surface, what fears have been keeping you stuck, what you're really craving, what keeps you anxious, and then allow Him to lead you back onto the right path.

God created us, and He knows us better than we know ourselves. Doesn't it make sense to seek Him for answers instead of trying to figure it out ourselves?

Self-Reflection

Your journey starts not with figuring out the right diet or workout program. That will come after. To move towards your goal, you will first need to identify why you keep making the same mistakes over and over again. Why are you always starting over? Why are you always on a diet? Why aren't you doing the things you know to do?

You may be saying to yourself:

- If only I was more disciplined
- It's my emotional eating
- I don't have enough time—my schedule is too busy
- If only I would exercise more
- If only I had a faster metabolism
- It's my sweet tooth

These all sound like valid reasons, but they are only the effect of a deeper cause, symptoms of a deeper issue. Like a check-engine light in the car that provides clues into what's really going on in order to fix the car, we've got to check out our engine (our thoughts).

Thoughts Drive Action

Our engines are our subconscious thoughts. They drive our actions. They keep us repeating the same behaviors over and over again. Unless you're a mechanic, you have no idea about the inner workings of a car; and in our case, our subconscious mind. You just know that something is off. The excess weight is our clue that something is off—that's our check-engine light.

Because we're not mechanics. We start tinkering around, making wild, random guesses about what the problem is. We try to control our carbs, exercise more, make ourselves be more disciplined, pray more, but as you can probably attest none of these changes last. Sure you may lose some weight, but it always seems to find you again.

Get to the Root

There's a deeper issue at play that goes beyond eating less and exercising more. Until you get to the root of this, you will continue to spin your wheels. You will continue to self-sabotage, get overwhelmed, feel frustrated, disappointed, and discouraged. You will continue to experience anxiety around losing weight, and that's why you will subconsciously keep doing things that keep sabotaging yourself.

It's a Spiritual Battle

If you feel like you're always taking one step forward and two steps back, recognize that losing weight is a spiritual battle. It requires peeling back the layers and recognizing the unmet needs in your life then inviting God to fill them.

Self-Reflection

A few powerful questions to ask yourself are:

- What am I really craving? What emotions/needs/feelings am I stuffing?
- What will really satisfy me?
- What do I need to surrender to the Lord?
- What am I unwilling to face?

Ask the Holy Spirit to give you insight into these answers. Pour your heart out to God and commit this process to Him. Before you try another diet or weight loss program, be sure to ask God to search you. He is faithful and He will give you the answers you seek.

Chapter One

Your Words and Weight Loss

Speak Life AND Death

"The tongue has the power of life and death, and those who love it will eat its fruit." (Proverbs 18:21)

I often quote Proverbs 18:21 as my go-to Scripture that stresses the importance of speaking positivity and blessings over myself. For me, it means that when you speak positively and affirmingly, you will reap the rewards. And conversely, when you speak negatively or in disempowering ways you will experience the negative consequences of your speech.

Then I met with my pastor the other day, he gave me a whole new perspective on this Scripture that I had never seen before. He pointed out that life and death are not necessarily good and bad—meaning speaking life to things is not always positive and speaking death is not always negative.

This got me to thinking seriously about some of the things I say that I have given life to. I realize that a lot of the things I've thought about—and, as a result, said—I have given life to when I should have killed them. I've allowed destructive thoughts, patterns, and mindsets to fester for too long. I've had conversations with girlfriends; I've orchestrated dramatic pity parties and replayed them like broken records for so long that they've taken up residence in my mind and become a part of my identity. Trouble is, they had no business even taking up space in my head let alone leaving my mouth.

I realize that I've been speaking life over things when I should have used the power to speak death over them instead. Things like:

- Speaking life into my weaknesses
- Speaking life into things that are not going the way I want them to
- Speaking life over my health issues
- Speaking life over my family challenges

The more I speak life over these areas, the more they expand. Instead, they need to be killed! I have the power to speak death over weakness, death over disappointment, death over poor health, and death over family crisis. I'm learning that every time I talk about my problems, I give them more life.

Until recently, I never considered the power of speaking death that Proverbs 18:21 teaches us. I recognize that in many areas, speaking the power of death can actually help me more than speaking life. When I speak death, I can stop strongholds from taking root in my life.

Using the analogy of a garden, "It's better to never allow weeds in the garden instead of wasting time every year constantly pulling them out—kill them right away before they take root."

God knows our propensity to keep tolerating what should not be tolerated; to keep compromising our standards and to keep moving our boundaries. That's why He gives us strict boundaries that He wants us to adhere to. He does not want us constantly trying to compromise and give in to temptations.

In 1 Samuel 15, God tells Saul to destroy ALL the Amalekites.

> *"You must completely destroy the Amalekites and everything that belongs to them. Don't let anything live; you must kill all the men and women and all of their children and little babies. You must kill all of their cattle and sheep and all of their camels and donkeys." (ERV)*

As harsh as it sounds, God knew the consequences of not totally wiping out our enemies. The Amalekites were relentless in their brutality towards the Israelites. They had no fear of God, and they were committed to harassing and plundering from the Israelites.

Unfortunately, not unlike us, Saul felt bad about destroying everything (2 Samuel 15:9), and again, like us, the result of not completely wiping them all out caused God to reject Saul as king, and also had generational consequences as the surviving Amalekites continued to pillage and plunder the Israelites.

The way I see it, Saul is no different from me (and maybe you, too). How many things has God said to kill? Not, 'try and see if it will work'; not 'pray about it and hope for the best'; not 'ask a friend for advice', but KILL. And yet you and I keep nursing and rehearsing it.

I don't know about you, but when I saw Proverbs 18:21 from this new perspective, I purposed in my heart to kill some things that I have kept alive that I should have put to death a long time ago.

I've been talking about some things, and thereby keeping them alive in my spirit that, effective immediately, I have decided to kill. I realize this doesn't make them just go away, but I release the hold they've had over my mind, emotions, and spirit. More specifically:

- There is the pain in my back that I keep talking about that, effective immediately, I have killed.
- There are things that I say about my husband that, effective immediately, I have killed.
- There is the language that I use about my ability to succeed in business that, effective immediately, I have killed.
- There are negative things that I say about myself every time I look in the mirror that, effective immediately, I have killed.

My tongue has the power of death, and I will use that power to kill the things that God has called me to kill. I will not allow them to take up space in my mind and life anymore.

It's an amazing feeling to no longer be held captive by your own words.

I invite you to also examine some of the words that you say and the language you speak, and to use your power in Christ to kill them today!

What are you ready to put to death?

Three Small Words You Should Never Say

"For as the body apart from the spirit is dead, so also faith apart from works is dead." (James 2:26 ESV)

Do you have faith?

I'm not talking about the kind of faith that believes in God. I'm talking about rock- solid faith that says, "no matter what, I trust You, Lord; no matter where You lead me, I will follow."

Faith that says, *"In your strength I can crush an army; with my God I can scale any wall."* (Psalm 18:29 NLT)

I truly believe that if you listen to someone long enough, you can learn a lot about their faith. The words we say reveal our faith *and* our fears. Our language tells the world whether we truly believe God's Word or if we're just giving it lip-service.

In our defense, we often don't realize how the things we say can sabotage our weight-releasing goals and keep us from receiving many of God's promises for us.

For example, there is one phrase that we say that always reveals our intentions (or lack of them). Even if we say we have rock-solid faith, when you use this phrase, it will give away what's really going on deep down inside. We're probably all guilty of using this phrase once, or 100 times. I often still catch myself saying it.

Let's look at it in the context of our health:

- "I need to get to the gym."
- "I need to eat better."
- "I need to lose some weight."
- "I need to spend more time in prayer."
- "I need to ...." (insert your need)

Regardless of how much faith you say you have, the phrase 'I need to' will keep you from achieving your weight releasing goals if you always use it.

Why?

- Because it focuses on what you lack, not your faith.
- It only serves as a reminder of what you're not doing (and probably will never do unless you develop a plan).
- It does not take God into account when you say it. It does not consider His strength, His grace, and His power to help you do the things that you are unable to accomplish in your own strength.
- Most importantly, it does not lead to action!

The Bible teaches us that faith without works is dead. So, my fellow overcomers, it's time to stop constantly rehearsing the phrase 'I need to', and actually do something!

'I need to' will never get you results. Saying 'I need to' will keep you in overwhelmed mode, in guilt mode, and in frustration mode. It will continue to erode your faith.

Never mind what you 'need to' do, what 'will' you do?

I'm not saying this is easy for you, but the Word teaches us that God's yoke is easy (Matthew 11:30). He will do the heavy lifting for us. He will do the things that we are unable to do in our own strength when we put our trust in Him. But it will take willingness on our part. We've got to take the first step in faith.

Change your language from 'I need to' to 'I will.'

Instead, say:

- "I will go to the gym on Saturday."
- "I commit to changing my eating habits by eating more vegetables."
- "I will achieve my goal weight by December 31st."
- "I commit to releasing weight by exercising for 30 minutes each day."
- "I will wake up 15 minutes earlier each day to pray."
- "I choose to stop eating dessert every day."

Note: You should always be specific and state the when, what, where, or how of the action you're committing to.

Can you see the difference between using words like 'commit', 'will', and 'choose,' instead of 'need to?'

When your mind receives the first few words, it sends a cue to take action, it feels inspired and ready to tackle the task, and it goes to work looking for solutions to solve the challenge.

But when your mind hears the words "I need to" (again):

- It gets overwhelmed with feelings of guilt for not doing what you know to do.
- It remembers all the times that you've attempted to do something and failed, so you will instantly get flooded with feelings of failure.
- It's like a form of mental procrastination. It may feel good temporarily to say it, but deep down inside

you're setting yourself up for a mental battle that you rarely win.

I challenge you today to get conscious of how many times you say the words "I need to."

It's very possible you might have just told yourself, "I need to read this section again so I can remember this" ... ha-ha.

Don't worry, change will take time. Start slowly with baby steps.

For now, don't try to stop yourself from saying it. Just ask the Holy Spirit to bring it to your awareness.

By the grace of God, you've got this!

Understanding the Power of Your Words in Your Weight Loss Journey

Words are so powerful that Psalm 33:6 states that, *"the Lord merely spoke, and the heavens were created."* (NLT) **If we are created in God's image, then is it possible that God has also given us this same power to create change with our words?**

Scripture says that we have also been given the power to speak to our situations and circumstances. *"… you could say to this mountain, 'Move from here to there, and it would move'"* (Matt. 17:20 NLT). How different would your life be if you began to speak powerfully to your situation in a proactive way that would cause it to change?

Proverbs 18:21 also teaches us that death and life are in the power of the tongue. This verse holds true whether we're speaking of spiritual, physical, or emotional 'life and death.'

Now take a moment and examine how you speak. When it comes to your health and your weight, do you speak negatively or positively?

You will NEVER reach your weight loss (or any other) goals if you're constantly saying words like:

- "It's hard"
- "I know, but…"
- "I want to"
- "I should"

- "I need to"
- "I don't know"

These words all speak of something in the future that will probably never happen, and they only keep you frustrated and procrastinating.

Your words precede action, and these words indicate inaction and failure.

Your words give the world a preview of what your true intentions or beliefs are about your ability to succeed.

Your words are so ingrained in you that you're often not even conscious of what you're saying.

Your words come out of your mouths on automatic pilot, and are subconsciously sabotaging your health and your lives.

Instead of speaking negatively about your body or your health, make verbal declarations about your health. I often share my personal declarations with my clients. Here is mine. I encourage you to create your own:

- I am in excellent health.
- I am in action every day to promote my health and the health of others.
- I create my health through my daily positive habits.
- I believe my health is important, and I strive to be in the best health.
- I attract healthy people, healthy attitudes, healthy food, healthy activities, and healthy habits into my life.
- My ability to be in better health increases day by day.

- I make time in my schedule every day for physical activity.
- I receive God's gift of excellent health. It allows me to serve in His Kingdom, to help more people, to enjoy a better quality of life, and to be free to worship.
- I weigh what God wants me to weigh, and I eat according to what God wants me to eat.
- I get plenty of rest each night.
- I have boundless energy.

As you go about your day, pay attention to how you speak to yourself. Are your words affirming or condemning? If they don't build you up, change them! Think of something you can say to yourself to reframe your negative comment. If you're complaining about the size of your hips, instead thank God for the ability to move every day!

Understanding the Power of Your Words in Your Weight Loss Journey - Part 2

Do you believe that your speech can impact your weight loss? I sure do. A big part of my coaching is to help women understand that their words precede their actions. So a good place to begin to change your negative actions is by changing your speech.

If your goal is to lose weight, here are 10 phrases to eliminate from your vocabulary:

1. **"It's Hard."** People often say exercise is hard—that making time for your health is hard. It's not hard—it's just new for you. But as you continue to tell yourself it's hard, your mind will come into agreement with your words and it will continue to get harder and harder for you.

2. **"I know."** People often say "I know." But the essence of truly knowing something is to do it. Until you do it, you don't really know.

3. **"But...."** Every time we say "but" we cancel out everything before the "but." When I tell someone to exercise for just 10 minutes a day I would hear, "I would love to exercise 'but' you don't know how hectic my schedule is." Essentially this means I really don't want to exercise.

"Gentle words bring life and health; a deceitful tongue crushes the spirit." (Proverbs 15:4 NLT)

4. **"I should"; "I want to"; "I must"; "I have to"; "I wish."** These are all future tense words that keep you procrastinating and making excuses. They only keep you stuck in the cycle.

5. **"I'll try."** This is another non-committal word. Use proactive, definite words that your mind will get excited about and find creative ways of obliging. Use words like, "I commit to" and "I choose to."

6. **"I'll start tomorrow or Monday."** The best time to start is now. Deferring your goal intensifies the perceived pain.

7. **"I don't know."** This phrase is equally as bad as "I know." It prevents you from thinking or taking action. If I ask someone when they plan on exercising and they respond with, "I don't know", it's a clear indication that they are not committed to their fitness program.

8. **"I can't."** People often will say, "I can't" even before they've tried. A more appropriate response is, "I will do my best."

9. **"I hate."** Clients say to me, "I hate cardio" or "I hate working my abs." The word hate has strong emotions tied to it, and like other words, when you say it enough it will become part of your subconscious mind which is beyond powerful. Instead, focus on the benefit of the activity you dislike.

10. **"I don't have the time."** This phrase is never the real issue. People who say they don't have the time have not made exercise a priority yet. You give your time to what you deem as important. If you are ready to get in shape, then you will make time.

Did you notice any of the words on the list that you say often? I challenge you to notice when you say them and start to replace them with something affirming instead—Scripture is always a great option, too!

Your words precede action, so if you're really ready to make a change in your health then it's time to get present to these words that you use and start to eliminate them from your speech.

"Wise speech is rarer and more valuable than gold and rubies." (Proverbs 20:15 NLT)

The Art of Learning to Say 'No'

"And don't say anything you don't mean. This counsel is embedded deep in our traditions. You only make things worse when you lay down a smoke screen of pious talk, saying, 'I'll pray for you,' and never doing it, or saying, 'God be with you,' and not meaning it. You don't make your words true by embellishing them with religious lace. In making your speech sound more religious, it becomes less true. Just say 'yes' and 'no.' When you manipulate words to get your own way, you go wrong." (Matthew 5:34-37 MSG)

Do you feel guilty when you tell someone 'no?' Or do you give someone a list of reasons why you're not able to say 'yes' to their request?

As Christian women, we were raised to be courteous, polite, giving, and gracious. Somewhere along the line, we took that to mean that we're to accept every request ever made. It's left many of us feeling overwhelmed and burned out.

Saying no stirs up a lot of guilt, awkwardness, anxiety, and fear of judgment from others.

We've been raised to believe that saying 'no' is selfish and self-centered.

As a recovering people-pleaser and over-giver myself, I've experienced negative effects of being afraid to say 'no.' I've been afraid to ask clients for fees even though I've fulfilled my end of our agreement. I've changed my schedule to accommodate others, even though it's a huge inconvenience to me. And I've even eaten foods I didn't want so I wouldn't offend people. After working with a coach and after much prayer, I'm learning how to overcome this stronghold.

What about you? What are some things that you've said 'yes' to when you really wanted to say 'no?'

Negative Impact of Not Saying 'No'

This pattern has such a negative impact on our overall health. We end up stuffing our feelings with food instead of speaking out. Why? It's one of the few things that gives us a sense of being in control. It's instant gratification that briefly soothes the stresses and feelings caused by not having maintained a healthy boundary. Ironically, we're actually out of control as our emotions are dictating our diet, and food will not cure a negative emotion, but excessive food will ultimately cause more negative emotions as our health and self-esteem suffer.

Not voicing our true feelings also causes a lot of stress in our bodies, which can result in a variety of stress-related illnesses ranging from high blood pressure, diabetes, depression, obesity, and gastrointestinal problems.

If you have trouble saying no, consider this ...

The Benefits of Saying 'No'

Frees up time and mental energy so you can say 'yes' to what's really important. How much of your time is spent doing things only because someone asked you, and not because you really wanted to? Consider this: You could be out of alignment with God's desire for you because you're afraid to say 'no.'

It will simplify your life and give you clarity. Life is really simple, yet we make it complicated by doing a lot of things that

God did not call us to do. Spend time with God and get clear on what He's called you to do, then learn to say 'no' to the rest.

It will give you peace of mind and decrease stress. Are you stressed because you've overextended yourself again? Maybe you're trying to keep up with the Joneses. Learning to say 'no' will create so much peace in your life because your focus will be on one thing, and one thing only, and that is pleasing God.

It gives you focus. Do you feel overwhelmed? Do you feel like your life is on a perpetual merry-go-round and it feels like you can never get off? Saying 'no' will help you focus on what's important while you learn how to leave the rest behind. Imagine waking up each day only having 3-4 items on your to-do list, and then ending your day with them completed. No distractions— no Facebook, no Candy-Crush, no unnecessary shopping or TV watching, nor giving people your time who do not respect it. Does that sound empowering?

Say no to:

- Anything not in alignment with your values
- Anything that will sabotage your health and weight loss goals
- The limiting beliefs that keep you stuck in the crazy cycle of losing and gaining weight
- Anything that steals your time and causes you to lose your focus
- Trying to please other people—focus only on what God thinks about you
- Obsessive weighing in on the scale or being hyper-focused on your weight
- Wasting time on social media sites, TV, gaming, or any time-suckers

- Blaming people
- Jamming your schedule with more to-do items than you know you have time for
- Giving your time to people who do not respect you or your time
- Foods that will keep you feeling sick and tired

Have a difficult time saying 'no?' Try these strategies:

1. It can be difficult to say 'no' to someone. Instead, say, "let me pray about it", "let me think about it", or "let me check my schedule." This will keep you from making a rash decision that you may regret.

2. Our nature is to underestimate how long something will take and overestimate our ability to do it. Whatever the request is, automatically double the time you think it will take, and then reconsider whether you really have enough time to do it.

3. Practice saying 'no.' This is a skill that everyone has to learn. Some people are better at it only because they've practiced more. Start in non-threatening areas and then graduate to more challenging ones. This might be work-related or with someone who has a hard time respecting boundaries.

Learning to say 'no' is not selfish. In fact, it is one of the most loving things you can do for yourself and others.

At first it will feel unnatural and intimidating, so instead of feeling the pressure of saying, "no" you might say,

- Let me pray about it
- Let me get back to you
- Let me sleep on it to be sure

Take time today to hear the voice of God in your schedule and your commitments. Get clear on what He's called you to do. Understand your assignment and purpose on this planet and use that as your guide to what you should and should not do. How is God leading you? He wants to be part of all of your decisions, so let Him in today.

Here's an example a friend of mine shared about her challenge with saying no:

> I spent six hours of my time driving someone to and from Orlando instead of asking them to leave their car at the airport. I could not do any work that day, and I need to work. My work is more important than driving someone who can take an Uber or leave their car at the airport. It is inconvenient for them, but they earn way more money than I do and can likely afford the parking fees. Losing a full day of work hurts financially, along with causing me to fall behind on my own priorities and responsibilities.

Can you see yourself in that example? What will you say 'no' to?

Chapter Two

Your Thoughts and Weight Loss

Transforming your Mind for Weight Loss

And do not be conformed to this world [any longer with its superficial values and customs], but be ʹtransformed and progressively changed [as you mature spiritually] by the renewing of your mind [focusing on godly values and ethical attitudes], so that you may prove [for yourselves] what the will of God is, that which is good and acceptable and perfect [in His plan and purpose for you].ʺ (Romans 12:2 Amp.)

As I'm writing this chapter, someone who is angry with me has chosen to write a very poor book review (although they have never read my books) in an attempt to 'get back at me for a wrong they feel I have caused them.' My flesh wants to lash out and get back at them for trying to malign my character. Then I read the scripture above and smiled.

You see, it's one thing to quote Scripture and praise the Lord, but it's quite another to put it into practice. It's one thing to say you trust God, but what do you do when your back is against the wall?

Romans 12:2 reminds us to mature spiritually, allowing God to change the way we think. So instead of lashing out at this person, I'm choosing to pray for him. I'm releasing him to God and asking Him to heal this person's brokenness. I'm asking God to show me what I need to learn in this situation instead of focusing on how I feel I've been wronged. And I will not pacify my feelings with food.

As you experience difficult situations in your life, do you conform by acting as the world acts, by worrying, obsessing about your situation, wallowing in self-pity, self-medicating with alcohol, food, or drugs? Do you try to take matters into your own hands? Or do you allow God to transform your thinking so that you can see the situation from His perspective?

In one of our courses in the WeightLossGodsWay.com program, we've been studying Romans 12:1-2. During our 6:00 a.m. call on Saturday, we took some time and reflected on situations that we were going through (including our weight loss journey), and we asked ourselves if we were conforming or transforming. Were we dealing with our problems the same way the world does, or were we allowing our situations to transform us?

Sometimes it can be difficult to see if we are practicing Godly principles during our trials, or to notice if we're acting the same as the rest of the world. Below is a list that we came up with.

Reflect on a situation that you are going through right now and ask yourself if you are conforming to the patterns of this world, or if you are being transformed by the renewing of your mind as Scripture directs us.

When we conform:

- We focus on the problem
- We are fixated on getting results now
- We complain and worry
- We focus on perfection
- We need to be in control
- We look for solutions from other people
- We set unrealistic expectations
- We make decisions based on fear and desperation
- We obsess about what others think about us and allow it to shape our decisions

When we transform:

- We focus on God ~ Heb 12:2
- We focus on God's timing, not ours ~ Ecc 3:1
- We trust and pray ~ Phil 4:6
- We focus on progress ~ 1 Cor 15:58
- We let God control the situation ~ Prov 19:21
- We ask God for His best solution ~ Rom 8:28
- We tell God our desires and leave the rest to Him ~ Ps 37:4
- We make decisions based on the Word of God ~ Heb 4:12
- We focus on what God thinks about us and who He says we are ~ 1 John 3:1

How Your Thoughts Affect Your Weight

I truly believe that renewing your mind is foundational to your breakthrough in your health and in all other areas of your life. Your battle with your weight is first lost or won in your mind, which must be renewed in order to conform to how God views things.

I realize that in order for me to continually renew my mind, I have to be aware of what's going on in there. I have to be conscious of my thoughts. I've realized that by the time I 'give in and eat something I did not plan', my thoughts had already been running roughshod in my mind and the damage was already done.

Many times, setbacks occur when we haven't planned ahead and we've let not only our minds, but our schedules, get off course. When we don't have both of these things under control, they can play off of each other and lead us into a downward spiral that can lead to stress-eating or going hungry for too long and then eating what is quick and easy. Then along comes a load of guilt upon our shoulders for getting off course, and there we go.

If you're anything like me and you live much of your life on automatic pilot, then you will have to learn how to increase your consciousness before the process of renewing your mind can be truly effective. If you're not sure if you live on automatic pilot then answer these questions below. If you know for sure that you need some help in this area then you can skip these questions and go right to action steps for developing your consciousness.

Conscious living (eating) is about choosing what you will eat instead of letting your mood dictate your diet. This means thinking about your decisions instead of being led by circumstances—like a hectic schedule, not being home for lunch, not packing a healthy lunch, and so on.

If you are not sure if you need to live more consciously, ask yourself the following questions. If you find yourself saying 'yes' to many of them, you might want to consider mastering this step before renewing your mind:

1. Do you plan what you're eating and the physical activity you do each day?

2. Do you eat what is put in front of you rather than foods you enjoy?

3. Do you find yourself stuck in an exercise rut or not exercising at all even though you really want to?

4. Do you find yourself overweight because you've been eating the same foods you've been eating for years?

5. Do you find yourself wasting time on Facebook or watching TV, hanging out with friends (or other activities), instead of exercising or doing things that contribute to your health?

6. Do you go through your days not thinking about what you're doing?

7. Do you find yourself wishing that you could do more or be more but instead just go with the flow of day-to-day life?

8. Are you in shock/disbelief/frustrated that you let your weight get so out of control?

If you answered "no" to all of these questions you're probably already living consciously, and you don't need this article at all. But for those who would like to live more consciously, read on.

How to Live Consciously

Living consciously is deceptively simple. It can change in one second and you may not even realize it. I'm going to outline as many strategies as I can think of. The goal is not for you to do them all right away but to see if any of them can be easily implemented into your life. Also pay attention to the ones that will have the biggest impact on your life and try them first.

1. **Wake up in prayer.** Before your feet hit the floor each morning, ask the Holy Spirit to make you conscious and aware of the traps and pitfalls that might sabotage you throughout the day. Learning to live consciously is a huge undertaking that will require more strength than we're capable of mustering up.

2. **Use your emotions as checkpoints.** Emotions such as anger, frustration, anxiety, sadness, loneliness, and tiredness may often lead us to eat. But what if we tuned in to those feelings instead of stuffing them? What if we changed the pattern of anger = eat, to anger = pray? I know it will not happen overnight, but if we continually apply this new paradigm instead of our old familiar pattern it will eventually lead to change.

3. **Pray throughout the day.** I admire the Muslim culture for their commitment to pray throughout the day. 'Salat' is the obligatory Muslim prayers, performed five times each day. Imagine if you took time out of your day, each and every day to (re)connect with God. How powerful would your life be? For me, I know that food would have less importance than it currently does.

4. **Set a goal each year.** Do you know what you want to accomplish this year for your health? There's a popular quote that says, 'A confused mind says no.' If you don't have a clear, consistent plan for your weight and health then your mind will say no to

it and default to whatever's comfortable. Do you have a clear and consistent plan for how to achieve it? Many of us are on automatic pilot because we have not taken stock of where we currently are and where we want to be.

5. **Consider the costs**. Many of us are not conscious of our thoughts around our health because we have not taken the time to consider the price we will have to pay to be in good health. There may be a financial investment of eating healthier foods, hiring a trainer, investing in exercise equipment, and maybe even seeking counseling.

You may need to sacrifice time that was devoted to other things, or you may need to wake up earlier to exercise, plan your meals, and plan your day. If something costs you then you will value it more and be conscious of your investment. I challenge you to take some time and write out all the costs associated with improving your health.

6. **Consider the consequences**. There are also consequences to inaction. When you take the time and realize that your poor health can lead to diabetes, high blood pressure, heart disease, strained relationships, inability to enjoy everyday activities, and so forth, then you will become more conscious on a daily basis of why a healthy lifestyle is so important.

7. **Take inventory.** There's a popular saying, "If you don't measure it, you can't manage it." A great exercise to do is to track what you do (and think). We do this exercise in our WeightLossGodsWay.com challenges and it's always so eye-opening, because it makes you aware of how much of your time is spent in negativity, procrastination, distractions, discouragement, and anxiety.

Try this tool—rescuetime.com—to help you track how you spend your time, or simply set an hourly alarm and check in on what you're thinking and doing every time your alarm goes off. Try this for 2–3 days to get a good picture of how you are doing.

8. **Saturate your mind.** I sometimes find myself singing along to popular songs in the car, only to realize that I'm singing about adultery, bondage, lust, desperation, 'gettin' down in the club,' and excessive drinking, and that's just the chorus. I know the lyrics because I hear them often; they get stuck in my head. So why can't we do the same thing with uplifting, empowering songs? I'm learning to play worship music as often as I can.

Post scripture all around your house, in your kitchen cupboards, on the dashboard of your car, in every mirror in your house, on your fridge. Remind yourself of God's word in all the places where you need to pay attention.

"For as he thinketh in his heart, so is he"
(Proverbs 23:7 KJB)

9. **Make time to disconnect.** For many of us, we don't take time to simply stop. We're on a non-stop hamster wheel that just keeps going and going. Taking the time to stop will completely throw off our entire schedule. But it's amazing what you'll learn about yourself and your Heavenly Father when you take some time to unplug and just be alone with yourself.

Many of us can't hear God talking to us because there's too much chatter and activity always going on in our minds and our lives in general. Last Sunday, I made a conscious choice to disconnect from everything and just 'be.' It was not stellar my first time around, but I know it will get better with time.

10. **Live in gratitude.** Years ago, I started a gratitude journal. This involves writing out 5 things you're grateful for each day. What starts to happen is that your mind will begin to search out and become more conscious of what you see, do, feel, and

think. Having hot water, feeling the sun shining, hearing birds singing, the ability to walk, see, read, and eat become activities to experience and cherish instead of daily mundane activities that we give no thought to.

Renewing your mind is a critical step for transforming your health and helping you lose weight, but first you have to learn how to take control of your thoughts. Are there any of these strategies you can put in place today? If you really want to renew your mind, then learn what currently has control of your mind and reclaim it as your own.

There's no quick fix or instant solution, but I promise you that if you learn how to renew your mind by first increasing your consciousness everything else will fall into place.

Your victory is at hand as you keep thinking about what you're thinking about.

Chapter Three

Your Emotions and Weight Loss

Emotional Eating—A Subconscious Response

Emotional eating is when we eat in response to our feelings, regardless of whether we're hungry or not. We can also use food as a tool or coping mechanism to either numb pain or to feel better. It's the automatic and subconscious responses that make our emotions so powerful and dangerous. At some point part of our brain may have initiated the sequence of events to eat, but then it became habituated and routine. When actions become habituated, they run on autopilot.

I remember when my doctor told me that I was borderline diabetic. You would think that would have been enough for me to change, but as much as I tried, I still could not stop myself from binging on sweets.

Why couldn't I stop, even though I knew this could lead to irreparable hardship? Because I was not conscious of what triggered my emotional eating. Even when I did gain awareness, willpower was no match for my feelings and emotions. I've spent most of my adult life learning how to stuff my uneasy feelings back down with food, so I don't have to feel them. Like a baby-soother or pacifier, a large population of society and I use food to comfort us. It makes us feel better when we're stressed, angry, lonely, bored, frustrated, or a multitude of other emotions that we experience.

But it's not supposed to be this way. Our goal is to learn how to **feel our feelings and feed our hunger** instead of feeding our feelings and refusing to feel hunger.

Feel Your Feelings

Why is it important to feel your feelings and feed your hunger? Because emotional eating plays a big factor in our "inability" to eat healthily and reach or maintain a healthy weight.

Experts estimate that 80% of overeating is emotional. I don't know who those experts are since this is one of those statistics that gets thrown around the health and wellness world, but my own life can attest to the relative accuracy. After my first meal of the day (around noon), most of what I eat is usually out of boredom, habit, anxiety. Or—if it's the weekend—entitlement.

My body feels healthiest when I eat a fairly large meal at lunch, a light snack a few hours later, followed by a very light meal around 5:00 P.M. Admittedly, everything outside of those three meals is emotional.

What's at the root?

Know this. There's a reason you choose to feed your feelings instead of feeling them, because these feelings are painful! Their roots are grounded in discomfort, pain, or trauma. And why on earth would we want to experience pain?

Except you probably know all too well that 'feeding' them with food does not take away the pain permanently. The benefit, if you want to call it that, lasts only as long as the taste of the food swirls around in your mouth. Soon after that comes the guilt and shame, if you're conscious of your patterns. If you're on automatic pilot, then you may not even be aware of why you're eating when you're not hungry.

In Ephesians 4:26-27, "Be angry, and yet do not sin; do not let the sun go down on your anger, and do not give the devil an opportunity."(SEV empathize added), Paul is using the emotion of anger, but we can apply any emotion that leads us to eat. He is saying that we can feel our feelings, but we don't have to act on the feeling. We can feel anger, frustration, sadness, or stress and **not** eat to numb those unwanted feelings. As we learn how to stop allowing our emotions to lead our behavior, we keep the enemy from having control of our health.

3 Keys to End Emotional Eating

I encourage you to pay attention to the emotions that dictate and sabotage your health. Then you'll discover how to let the Word of God dictate your actions, choices, decisions, and behaviors. It's the only way to true healing and freedom.

Just for today, track everything you eat. Write it in a journal, placing either an "H" for hungry or "E" for emotional beside everything you eat. If you're not hungry, assume it's emotional.

Then write out what the emotion is that led you to eat. See what you discover about your eating habits.

1. Courage to Feel

Most people who eat emotionally do so to escape negative emotions they don't want to feel. So healing starts with taking an honest look at your eating behavior. Keep a food journal and pay attention to those times when you are eating when you aren't hungry. What is the emotion that you are feeling? Is it anger, depression, boredom, stress, unworthiness?

Whatever the emotions are, you must have the courage to stop burying them under food and face them.

2. Willingness to Trust

Once you identify the emotions, you need faith to believe that you can handle them with God's help. In Psalms 46:1, you are assured that God is your refuge and strength, a very present help in trouble.

When I dealt with emotional eating, I used food as a substitute for God. So, one of my first steps was to be willing to let go of my dependence on food and grab hold of God during emotional storms. It was the best decision I ever made, not only in my health but in my peace of mind.

3. Allowing God's Power to Work Within You

Ephesians 3: 20 says: *"Now to Him who is able to do exceedingly abundantly above all that we ask or think, according to the power that works within us."* (NKJV) You have power inside you to change! If you have accepted Jesus Christ as your Savior then you have the Holy Spirit living inside you, which is the same power that raised Jesus from the dead.

The enemy deceives many into believing they are helpless victims with no power.

- He wants you to believe that you will never change.
- He doesn't want you praying.
- He doesn't want you praising God for what you have.
- He doesn't want you meditating on the excellencies of God.
- And he especially doesn't want you studying God's Word!

He knows that once you start doing those things, the power working within you will grow and you will no longer be open to his destructive suggestions. You will find that the comfort you were seeking is obtained best when you rely on God rather than food.

Through practicing spiritual disciplines like prayer, praise, worship, and study of God's Word regularly, food will begin to resume its proper place in your life and God can assume His proper place: First in all areas.

How Feelings of Rejection Impact Your Weight Loss

I woke up the other morning from a very vivid dream. As I think about it now, I can feel the bitter sting and pain as it took me back to a familiar childhood memory—one of rejection.

In my dream, one of the women at my church rejected me by inviting the 'popular' group of women to her party and boldly told me that I was not welcome. I remember the look of disgust on her face as she told me that she did not like me.

As I sought the Lord about my dream (which is something I just started doing), He showed me what the dream was about. A couple of days before the dream, my husband said something to me which I thought was very hurtful. He said it as a thoughtless pondering and did not mean any harm by it. Even though he apologized, it sat with me for days. I ruminated on it, obsessed about it, and replayed his words in my head until I crafted a song in my mind to make sure I remembered his words!

The Holy Spirit showed me that my dream about being rejected was at the root of why my husband's words hurt so badly. His seemingly insignificant comment took me back to a string of rejections from an ex-husband, from my son's father, best friends, boyfriends, and my own father's abandonment when I was a child. All of these events changed me; they redefined how I see people and how I see myself. They confirmed a lie that the enemy whispered in my ear at some point, and I believed it.

When many of us experience rejection as a child it's as if we are given a pair of tinted glasses which we begin to wear, and from that point on everything we experience looks and feels like rejection.

Have you ever felt the sting of rejection? It hurts bad, doesn't it? That's why we keep it buried deep, so it does not rear its embarrassing and sobering head. Except, it does rear its head. It comes out in various ways. When someone gives us their opinion, we take it as rejection. When someone refuses our suggestion, we take it as rejection. And when someone does not include us, we take it as rejection regardless of the intent behind it.

So, what does rejection have to do with our health?

Many of us eat and we don't even know why we're eating. We just know we 'need' something, and we need it bad. Many of us never make the connection back to the feeling we experienced earlier on in the day, when we thought someone was talking about us, or when we're not included in what we thought should have been an important decision. Instead of expressing these feelings, we stuff them deep down inside. But here's the problem—feelings are meant to be felt, not fed!

Something may happen to throw our emotions off in the morning, but later in the day, when we're now in the privacy of our own homes, the feelings may well up again. But this time we've got the luxury of food to help stuff them back down. This is the cycle so many of us repeat each day. This cycle is what keeps so many of us overweight and out of touch with our feelings.

We eat instead of confronting our spouses, for fear of rejection. We eat after a stressful day at work when people got on our last nerve but we did not confront them, for fear of rejection. We eat instead of speaking up at church and end up taking on more than we can manage, for fear of rejection. We eat instead of saying no when a friend or coworker asks us to do something we don't want to do, for fear of rejection. We can even eat when we are pressured to eat by those around us at a social gathering, for fear of rejection.

It gets so chronic that we often just eat and don't know why we're eating. But what if we were to take the time and seek the Holy Spirit, instead of searching for some other means of feeling full and taking away our sadness, guilt, frustration, or fear? He will not only show us what's at the root, but also give us a solution. We simply need to ask Him to show us what to do.

As I woke up from my dream, I was blessed by a colleague's post about rejection (takebackyourtemple.com/dont-fooled-rejection/). I praise God for His timing, because it ministered to that broken place in me.

Here are four strategies that I learned as a result of my experience, and my time in prayer. I pray that they are a blessing to you, too.

1. Commit to Go Deeper

The next time you feel the desire to eat when you're not hungry, ask the Holy Spirit to show you what's at the root of this desire. Trust and wait for the answer. My dream occurred two days after the comment from my husband, but it was clear that it was God talking to me. My answer from Him was to 'take off my rejection-tinted glasses and see the world and my experiences from God's perspective.'

If you don't know where to begin with going deeper, I encourage you to spend some time and meditate on this scripture in Psalms 139:23: *"Search me, God, and know my heart; test me and know my anxious thoughts."* The answer may not come right away, but I promise you it will come.

Another verse to consider is 1 John 3:16. *"This is how we know what love is: Jesus Christ laid down his life for us."*

As people-pleasers, we can waste so much time worrying over what others think of us. What we really need to focus on is how much God loves us. When we are seeking to please God only—an audience of one—and we know in our hearts that we are doing our best to please Him and walk by faith, why should we concern ourselves with anyone else's approval?

Sure, people's words may hurt. Disappointment may sting. But we can grow thicker skins as we start ignoring negative comments, praying to be positive when life gets us down, and focusing our minds on the positive promises yet to come and be fulfilled in our lives. God never promises a bump-free ride in life. But He does promise to get us to the promised land at the end of our journey. We are so blessed to be loved and forgiven. Let's focus on this permanent truth, and not so much on the temporary frustrations of life.

2. Commit to the Process

Many of us wear our scars like proud tattoos, even when we know what's at the root. I made up a song to my husband's words so that I could remember the pain of rejection. Why do we romanticize our pain? Why do we need to feel like a victim? My theory: It's what we know. It's comfortable to us because we've lived with it for so long. Experiencing anything other than rejection would contradict our song that we've been singing for so long. We know that song very well.

But what if we learned a new song? One that didn't have the lyrics of a sad country song? What if we learned the lyrics to Pharell's song, 'Happy?'

Psalms 147:3 teaches us that there is healing for us. We can take our brokenness to God, and He can and will restore us to wholeness. It's necessary to experience the abundant life that Christ died for us to have, but we've got to commit to it.

Most of us want to bypass this stage. We just want to get to the good parts. Unfortunately, there are no shortcuts. We've got to put in the time.

Like peeling back the layers of an onion there's always more that we discover about ourselves, especially as God brings us to higher levels in Him. We must strip away all of this dead weight if we truly want to be free.

"He heals the brokenhearted and binds up their wounds."
(Psalms 147:3)

3. Commit to Forgive

Forgiving my husband for his comments was the easy part. Then I heard the Holy Spirit ask me, 'Have you forgiven your ex-husband?' 'Your son's father?' 'Your own father for leaving you?' 'Have you forgiven yourself for believing that everything that happened to you was somehow your fault?' Forgiving my wrong-doers and myself...not so easy. Especially when the pain of their hurts have a lasting impact on my future.

For many of us, we have to live with the consequences of past actions for the rest of our lives. Without healing and forgiveness, other people's mistakes will affect our future, our health, and our perspective on life. Without the inner working of the Holy Spirit, we will live in continual suffering from the sins of others and continue to see the world with the tinted glasses of rejection on.

"And when you stand praying, if you hold anything against anyone, forgive them, so that your Father in heaven may forgive you your sins." (Mark 11:25)

We also need to remember that forgiveness is also about our own healing; emotionally, mentally, and physically. It's been scientifically proven that holding on to anger, bitterness, resentment, anxiety, and fear can lead to disease and distress within the physical body. Headaches, stomachaches, irritable bowel syndrome, physical pain, and many other symptoms are listed as side-effects of not dealing with these types of issues.

Let's let go of past hurts and forgive and go on to being healed in every area of our lives.

4. Commit to Love

As the Holy Spirit ministered to me as I awoke from my dream, these words that I once heard at a conference came into my thoughts: **"I am loved lavishly by God."** I repeated it over and over that morning.

I emphasized the word "I" first, then "loved," then "lavishly," then "God." God loves me lavishly. Me? I said it until I actually started believing it. Then even more, until I was convinced of it. Then even more, until I was able to get myself out of bed and start my day without the sting of my dream, my husband's comment, and the weight of all the memories that attached themselves to it.

Now, as I look through the fridge and forage through the cupboards my thought is often, "What feelings am I trying to stuff?" To which my answer is often anger, frustration, or rejection. I then ask God to fill me with His love. When you know that God truly loves you, then you can believe and receive all of His promises and believe that they are for you. When you know that God truly loves you, then you can begin to love yourself by taking care of your body AND not accepting rejection as your theme song or keeping it on the replay cycle.

I pray God's peace and blessing over you as you take off your rejection-tinted glasses and see yourself as your Heavenly Father sees you: healthy, whole and lavishly loved!!!

Managing Disappointment in Your Weight Loss Journey (How to Overcome the Disappointment Cycle)

One of the comments I hear used by clients most often is, *"I'm so disappointed in myself!"*

Over the years of working with clients, disappointment is one of the most frequently experienced emotions and states that we experience on our weight loss journey.

Disappointment is the feeling you experience in the pit of your stomach when things don't turn out as you expect them to.

As frustrating as this constant feeling might be in your life, it is your body's way of getting your attention. This pain of disappointment is what gets you to eventually take the action needed to do something to relieve the pain. You see, our brains are always looking for ways to feel good. Unfortunately, instead of taking concrete action to dissipate the disappointment we sometimes substitute other things that make us feel good (or that taste good) instead.

What's more unfortunate is that our need to always feel good is what leads us into a vicious cycle of constantly gaining and losing weight.

Here's how it works:

When you experience a disappointment like stepping on the scale, having someone criticize you, or scraping your knee, your body releases cortisol. This is a stress hormone that alerts you to 'do something now' to get rid of the pain.

To eliminate the pain, your brain goes into its past memory files and recounts experiences that made you feel better in the past. So if your mom or dad gave you a popsicle when you scraped your knee when you were five years old then your brain will make a positive connection that says: pain = bad, treat = good, so pain = treat.

Your brain likes old memories, even when they lead you down the wrong path. That's because these well-worn, familiar pathways give you feelings of control and safety. Every time you experience this happy feeling from your childhood memories your body releases endorphins, which are hormones that make you feel happy. This endorphin release comes from two places. 1: the happy memory of your childhood, and 2: The sugar in the popsicle.

This 'pain = treat' connection remains with us into adulthood. However, with overuse we become accustomed to the endorphin release from the same stimulus. But rather than finding new sources of being happy, we just use more of the same. We eat/shop/drink/gamble more. Many of us continually try to get constant happiness from food, but not only are the returns depreciating but the overuse leads to being overweight. Which leads to disappointment, which leads to seeking the cure for disappointment, which the brain says is still more food. Too much of a good thing always becomes a bad thing.

*"Have you found honey? Eat only what you need, that you
not have it in excess and vomit it."* (Proverbs 25:16)

So why don't we just find new ways of being happy? It's not
that easy. While forming these kinds of associations was simple
as children, in our adult brains we may have zero reference for
exercise being pleasurable but tons of past experiences saying
ice cream is pleasurable. Not only does our subconscious mind
resist the attempt to find a different, unknown, unconfirmed
path to happiness, but it'll use the trick that it knows will get
you back on what it considers the 'right' path—disappointment.
We often undermine our own best intentions so we can stay
disappointed and continue to get our end 'hit' of pleasure-
inducing ice cream (or whatever we learned to use to feel better).

So just how do you overcome this cycle?

1. **Understand what's at the root of your feelings of
    disappointment.** Remember, our body is giving us
    cortisol not to eat more but for us to take action on
    that which is causing us discomfort. So, identifying
    what the REAL source of disappointment/discomfort/
    stress is gives us a clue as to what action needs to be
    taken. Sometimes there is no action that can be done
    at present, but knowing the real source can help us
    to choose more productive and healthy ways to get
    out of feeling disappointed.

    Often, the disappointment is caused by our imagined
    fears and not an actual circumstance. For example,
    if you've accepted the belief that you're unlovable as
    a child, even in adulthood you may act accordingly,
    either being defensive or reclusive around others,
    which isolates us, which leads to feelings of
    disappointment (as we 'prove' our fear is valid).
    Even if there is no actual circumstance, just the

expectation that one will happen can keep us feeling disappointed. Once you become familiar with the faulty thought patterns and limiting beliefs that your mind is defaulting to, then you can begin to work on the real problem.

2. **Renew your mind with the Word of God.** As you learn the root causes of your feelings, the next step is to begin to reprogram and renew your mind through the Word of God. God calls us to see the world from His perspective and not through our own limiting beliefs and thoughts. So, when those false beliefs bring us into disappointment, we can declare God's truth over them and break their hold over us.

3. As you get present to the root of the problem and renew your mind, the final and crucial step is to **practice new healthy habits**. Otherwise, our subconscious will continue to remain in the familiar feelings and situations.

Weight Loss Tips for Stressful Times

A few years ago, I was going through a very difficult time. Although I smiled and kept on going, as any good stoic Christian girl would, my body could not hide my stress. I started eating lots of junk—to the point where I had become borderline diabetic. I was exhausted all the time, and despite all my crazy workouts, I was steadily gaining weight. Mentally, I felt like I was in a perpetual brain fog. I found it difficult to concentrate, so Netflix became my best friend. I would binge-watch shows for 8 to 10 hours at a time!

Thankfully those days are now few and far between. My blood sugar is normal, my energy is high, and I can't remember my last serious Netflix binge.

Do you find it difficult to stay on track and keep losing weight during stressful times in your life? You're not alone. So many women share that they do well when life is going smoothly, but as soon as stress hits them it's their health that suffers.

Here are three big mindset shifts that you can make to help you remain healthy during stressful times.

1. Rethink Your Perspective on Health

Many of us have our health and weight loss in a category with cleaning the house, calling up an old friend, or even reading the Bible more. It's one of those things that we know we 'should do', we 'want to do it more', and 'wish that' we were more consistent at it. We really want to do it, but we're so busy that it never seems to make our priority list.

Instead of thinking of your health and weight loss as something you should do, think about it in the following ways:

See your health and fitness as the best antidepressant ever created.

- Instead of seeing health as another thing to check off your to-do list, see it as a necessity for life. Just like brushing your teeth every day and taking a shower, see your health as one of your daily habits.

- Understand that the more stressful life gets, the more you will need to eat well and exercise. This is the first thing we drop when we get stressed, but if we really understood its value, we would actually exercise more when we're stressed, not less.

When we're stressed, we sometimes want to lie on the couch and do nothing or eat some junk food to give us temporary relief. The next time you're feeling stressed, do the opposite of what you might normally do. Do something to improve your health—drink some water, go for a walk, eat some fruits or vegetables.

2. Rethink Your Perspective on Time

How many of us wished we had more time in the day? How many times have you said, "I'm soooo busy?" And lastly, how many of us have no time or energy to maintain our health and fitness program?

A lot of our frustration and stress arises because we're doing things that God never called us to do. We do them because we feel pressure from others, we think it's the right thing to do, or we do it for acceptance and approval. Unfortunately, this only leaves us feeling worn out and stressed out.

Here are a few tips to rethink your perspective on time:

- There are 24 hours in a day, Evaluate the priorities that God has called you to do and leave the rest. It won't be easy, but it's the only way to maximize your time.

- Stop trying to prioritize your schedule. Instead, schedule your priorities and make sure that your health is always one of them.

- There will never, ever, ever be enough time in one day to get everything done. No matter how we do today, no matter how productive we are, we will never get it all done. When we can understand that, then we can go to bed each day believing that we've done our best instead of feeling guilty and regretful that we did not get it all done.

- Lack of time is usually a problem of overcommitting, poor focus, or wasting time. Can you see how you waste some of your time? Is it playing internet games, watching TV, or surfing social media?

A lot of our stress is self-induced because of our inefficient or ineffective use of time. Take an inventory of how you spend your time to see if there are areas that you can tighten up so you can use your time more efficiently. Pray for wisdom for how you can do this (Psalms 90:12).

3. Rethink your Perspective on Control

This is one of my go-to scriptures in the Bible: *"What causes fights and quarrels among you? Don't they come from your desires that battle within you?"* (James 4:1). Why? Because it cuts right to the core of why I'm often so stressed out and frustrated.

My wants, my desires, my need to be in control is often in conflict with God's best for me. God wants me healthy for a variety of reasons, but maintaining my health and weight may not always be convenient for me. It takes me out of my comfort zone sometimes, and messes up my plans and takes sacrifice, which, let's face it, is not pleasant.

But here's the truth about control:

- The more we try to control things, the less in control we actually feel.

- One of the most stressful things we can do is to try to hold it all together and act like we have things all figured out.

- The more stressful life gets, the more we need to surrender control to God.

God calls us to rest in Him, **especially** during stressful times. So why do we continually try to maintain control?

"Come to me, all you who are weary and burdened, and I will give you rest." (Matthew 11:28)

Life would be so much more peaceful if we stopped trying to be all, do all, and handle it all, and surrender to our Heavenly Father. Ask yourself right now if God call you to do the things you did today? If you're struggling with your health and weight because you're so stressed and busy, I encourage you to spend some time in prayer and ask the Holy Spirit to give you a fresh perspective on your health, your time, and your need for control.

Weight Management and Depression

A few weeks ago, during one of our Seek Him Saturday calls, one of our members brought up the topic of depression.

To my surprise, more than 60% of the women on the call also struggled with depression. Since then, I've been hearing story after story about the 'dark cloud' that seems to permeate every single area of some women's lives—including their weight loss.

Whether you suffer from bouts of depression or full-blown paralysis where you're not able to get out of bed, you already know that it impacts your weight.

They are so intertwined because the part of the brain responsible for emotion—the limbic system—also controls appetite, so what affects one will usually affect the other.

It's difficult enough losing weight, but now attempt to do it when you have no will, desire, or motivation.

I'm no doctor or psychiatrist, but I will share a number of prescriptions that come from working with hundreds of women over the years. Try one or more, and be sure to give yourself lots of grace and patience.

Tips for Weight Management and Depression

Recognize that some days will be better than others. Maximize the great days by focusing on eating nutritious foods and moving your body, and pray through the challenging days. Not every day will be great. If you have that expectation then you'll always be disappointed, which can further your depression. Pray for wisdom. Ask the Holy Spirit to show you when you need to push through and make time for exercise and when you need to rest.

Although **exercise and healthy eating** might be the last things that you want to do, **recognize that they will help with both your depression and your weight.** Even going for a walk and getting some fresh air will help lift your spirit. When you exercise your body releases endorphins, which interact with receptors in your brain to make you feel better. They act as an analgesic, which diminishes the perception of pain.

Turn your worries and fears into prayers. I've heard it said that, *"If you can worry, then you can pray."* It's the same process of repeating a thought over and over in your mind. As you experience anxiety, worry, or feeling blue, turn those feelings into prayers and let God know that you need Him in whatever situation you're worried about.

Seek professional help if necessary. Many people believe that Christians should not be depressed. That's like saying, "Christians should not get cancer." Whether or not you think we should or should not, WE DO! Knowing something is 'off' in your mind needs just as much attention as knowing something is 'off' in your body, so seek treatment if your depression is affecting your daily activities.

Live in gratitude. It's hard to find something to be grateful for when everything is tainted with a dark cloud. Philippians 4:6-7 tells us, *"Do not be anxious about anything, but in every situation, by prayer and petition, with thanksgiving, present your requests to God. And the peace of God, which transcends all understanding, will guard your hearts and your minds in Christ Jesus."*

Turn each day over to the Lord and ask Him to order your day. We're constantly trying to fix ourselves and doing things that God has not called us to do. This can cause a lot of stress, anxiety, and frustration. Before you start each day, ask God what He wants you to focus on. Pray for strength for the day and eat healthily; make good decisions and be in His will. *"You will make known to me the path of life; In your presence is fullness of joy; In Your right hand there are pleasures forever."* (Psalm 16:11)

Find other ways to feel better instead of turning to junk food. Here's the vicious cycle: You feel depressed, so your body craves sugary and fatty foods to make you feel better, you temporarily feel better, then quickly feel worse, so you feel more depressed and the cycle continues. Choose foods that will boost your mood instead. Choose foods such as dark chocolate, nuts, seeds, avocados, and apples, to name a few.

Go deeper. Don't focus on trying to make yourself feel better. Depression is a symptom of a deeper cause, be it physiological, behavioral, psychological, nutritional, or spiritual. Get to the root of your depression instead of focusing on the symptoms.

Connect with others. There is a real enemy out there, and his assignment is to steal, kill, and destroy. He knows that when he can isolate you alone with your thoughts, he will win. This applies to both depression and overeating. Create a proactive plan and let friends and family know that if they have not heard from you in a while to contact you. Ask them to pray for you, and tell them what you will need from them to help you through those difficult times.

Establish a routine. Depression can take structure from your life. Establishing a routine can provide much-needed structure, which can help you feel safe and in control. Be sure to include morning prayer, listening to motivational music, and walks in your routine.

Note: This post is in no way intended to treat depression. It's to help women whose depression is getting in the way of their weight loss progress. If you're battling depression or experiencing suicidal thoughts, please seek professional care.

Chapter Four

Your Behavior and Weight Loss

How Perfectionism is Sabotaging Your Weight Loss

A shout-out to all the perfectionists out there! You know who you are!

- It drives you crazy to see a typo in the article or post you're reading.
- You'll spend hours working on something until you get it just right.
- You can't stand when things are not neat and orderly.
- You've been known to iron your bedsheets.

There are a lot of worse things you could be, right? Of course, but did you know that a spirit of perfectionism also sabotages your weight loss goals?

See if you recognize any of these patterns:

- You spend time and money coming up with the proper strategy to lose weight but never take action or stick with it.
- You're always "getting ready to get ready", but again have trouble with execution.
- Health becomes another stress as you can get caught up counting calories and tracking instead of focusing on the actual goal of losing weight.
- You can get obsessive about eating and exercising.
- You can go from the extreme of being disciplined to binging, and as a result you don't stick to your plan.
- You set unrealistic weight-loss goals and standards.
- You beat up on yourself a lot.

Any of these sound familiar? If so, the solution is to understand what's at the root of your perfectionism, and the answer may surprise you.

It's fear!

Yes, deep down inside perfectionists fear that they are not good enough, and feel like they are unable to please anyone—including themselves, so they just keep trying harder and harder.

A healthier approach is to understand that although God does call us to walk in excellence, it is different from perfectionism. Perfectionism says, "I must be the best." Whereas excellence says, "I want God's best for my life."

Practice creating realistic expectations instead of setting unachievable "realistic" goals. But even deeper than your goals is your need to understand God's gift of grace, and know that He loves you and accepts you just the way you are.

Fear shows up in our health and weight releasing journey in so many ways. It looks like procrastination, excuse-making, blaming, and even illness! But once you understand how fear shows up for you, then you can learn to let it go and give it over to God.

How a Spirit of Rebellion Can Prevent You from Reaching Your Weight Loss Goals

What is a spirit of rebellion?

How do you know you have one?

Maybe you're just unmotivated or you're just 'strong-willed?' Could this be a part of what keeps sabotaging your weight loss goals?

We've all heard of the rebellious teenager who starts cutting classes or the rebellious child that refuses to eat their vegetables. In fact, we all tend to have a bit of a rebellious streak in us—it's part of our sinful nature.

But what happens when that childhood or teenage rebellion continues into adulthood and impacts various areas of your life, especially your ability to lose weight?

Is it even possible that a rebellious spirit can be blocking your weight loss success? Take this little quiz and see if you identify with any of these scenarios:

1. You have a fight or disagreement with someone, but instead of telling them how you really feel you rush home so you can stuff your feelings with food?
2. You get close to your goal weight and then start to sabotage yourself.

3. You tell yourself that it's not fair that other people get to eat whatever they want, so you eat like they eat even though you know the consequences.

4. You clearly hear God directing you to take a certain action yet, like Jonah, you take another course of action.

5. You eat in secret.

If you're nodding your head in agreement, keep reading. Your deliverance is about to come!

"For rebellion is as the sin of witchcraft..."
(1 Samuel 15:23 KJB)

First off, there's a difference between 'being rebellious' (which we all are from time to time) and having a 'spirit of rebellion' (or rebellious spirit).

A rebellious spirit is a stronghold that continually controls your actions. It is argumentative (either passively or outwardly); it resists authority and often thinks it knows best, or it doesn't feel like doing it any other way. It does not like to be told what to do.

Unless the spiritual root of rebellion is addressed, it will continue to block your development, deliverance, or freedom from your weight loss as well as other areas of your life.

For many of us, our rebellious spirit that was developed in our childhood came about as a defensive mechanism, as a result of some kind of rejection, or deep emotional hurt. It may have been our only sense of power when we felt powerless.

Due to painful circumstances, you may have made up your mind that no one is going to force their will on you, or you may have learned how to comfort yourself with food to escape the pain. Rebellion was your only internal weapon of choice.

Your rebellious spirit that protected you as a child now shows up in the most unwanted and inconvenient ways as an adult. It will 'force' you to overeat or dishonor your body as a way to get back at someone or something and make you feel like you are in control.

The irony is that it's the spirit of rebellion in you that's in control and not actually you yourself. So, your attempts to be in control actually have you out of control. This leads to shame, guilt, disgust, and disappointment, and so the cycle continues.

The Solution for a Rebellious Spirit

The solution for rebellion is simple in principle yet difficult to put into practice, and that's why so many of us are stuck.

1. **Call a spade a spade.** It's a lot easier to call myself an emotional eater or even blame it on my low blood sugar than to say I have a rebellious spirit, but this will never bring about my deliverance.

You must understand what spirit you're dealing with in order to pray against it and cast it out. Admit that your rebellious spirit is what has been sabotaging you and keeping you from being in total communion with God.

2. **Repent.** 1 John 1:9 says: *"If we confess our sins, He is faithful and just to forgive us our sins and cleanse us of all unrighteousness."* (ESV) God is not mad at you; He won't punish you for not putting 100% of your faith and trust in Him, but you will miss out on your blessings. Unless we repent, though, we are tying God's hands and He cannot do what He wants to do in your life. Right where you are … right now … repent against your spirit

of rebelliousness and let God know that you want Him to be the Lord of your life.

3. **Submit.** Galatians 5:16 says, *"But I say, walk by the Spirit, and you will not gratify the desires of the flesh"* (ESV) **and** James 4:7 says, *"Submit yourselves, then, to God. Resist the devil, and he will flee from you."* **Satan has no access to us when we are walking in the Spirit and submitted to God.**

I believe that submission is a moment-by-moment choice. Start your day in prayer, end your day in prayer, and as often as you can remember throughout the day to continually turn everything you do over to God. Definitely spend a moment in prayer before you put anything in your mouth or consider doing anything that will negatively affect your health.

4. **Renew your mind.** Romans 12:2 says: *"Do not conform to the pattern of this world, but be transformed by the renewing of your mind. Then you will be able to test and approve what God's will is-- his good, pleasing and perfect will."*

Even though we have been renewed after repenting, our mind (speech and actions, too) may take a while to catch up. We must make a conscious effort of continuous renewal of our mind by guarding what we read, who we talk to, and what we say about ourselves. Equip yourself with scriptures to confess when you're feeling defeated.

5. **Do a new thing.** Although you've made room for God to do His part, you must also do your part to bring forth your deliverance from this spirit of rebellion.

What practical steps do you need to put in place to deal with this besetting sin? Do you need to take a course in assertiveness training? Do you need to change careers? Do you need to forgive those who have hurt you? Do you need to spend more time in prayer? Maybe you need to go to counseling?

Although it may not have been your fault as far as why you developed this spirit of rebellion, now that you know, it's your responsibility to do something about it. It's time to do something new so that you can begin to learn new habits and skills.

Beloved, remember that this weight loss journey has very little to do with the number on the scale. The number is just a physical manifestation of what's going on inside. If you desire permanent weight loss, get healing from the inside first. Get to the root of why you do what you do.

> " See, I am doing a new thing! Now it springs up; do you not perceive it?" (Isaiah 43:19)

You are blessed!

How to Overcome the Spirit of Guilt in Your Weight Loss Journey

There are so many different strongholds that keep us from achieving our healthy weight.

- The spirit of overwhelmedness.
- The spirit of perfectionism.
- The spirit of procrastination.
- The spirit of peoplepleasing.
- And the spirit of guilt.

First off, let's clear the air on a word that I use often—spirit. Why do I call it a spirit?

1. The Bible refers to this type of stronghold as a spirit (Eph. 6:11-19; 2 Tim. 1:7).

2. To help us recognize that it is something stronger than just our everyday normal feelings.

3. To help us understand the magnitude of these strongholds and recognize how they can take over our minds, bodies, and spirits just as an 'actual' spirit can.

For the record, I'm not well enough versed in theology to call these demonic spirits, but I can say that they are debilitating and powerful enough to keep you from fulfilling the destiny that God has on your life—from living in the joy, peace, and freedom that Christ died for us to experience. And more importantly, they can be **cast out** using the same biblical weaponry (Ps. 4:23; 1 John 3:20; 2 Cor 10:4).

Now that I've explained that (at least in my own mind,) let's move on to the topic at hand—GUILT.

Do you struggle with a spirit of guilt?

Let's check ...

- Are you constantly breaking your eating boundaries and then feeling guilty about it?
- Do you feel guilty when you have to tell someone 'no?'
- Are you always feeling guilty because you feel like you did not do enough, give enough, try harder, or love more?
- Do you find it hard to relax because you feel guilty and feel like you should be doing something else?
- Do you have a hard time enjoying anything like your home, car, finances because you feel guilty that you have more than others?
- Can you even remember the last time you did not feel guilty about one thing or another?

If you can identify with any of these, you probably struggle with a spirit of guilt.

Well, today is your day to lose that spirit from your life.

Why we feel guilty

Nothing good can ever come out of feeling guilty. Here are some of its lies:

- Guilt says that you are not worthy; not valuable enough to claim any of God's promises.

- It tells us that we do not deserve God's grace, but instead should feel bad whenever we miss the mark.

- It's our flesh's way of doling out self-punishment; it's like a really bad self-help tool.

- Guilt is a feeling that tries to control you into taking action, but feelings are not reliable sources of motivation or inspiration. Feelings are, well, just feelings, that can change moment by moment.

- Guilt temporarily takes away your responsibility by making you feel bad about what 'you should have' done (or not done) but it will never move you to action. In fact, it continues to sink you deeper into the pit of self-flagellation, shame, and doubt, which in turn causes you to turn to food to feel better, which then makes you feel even more guilt. What a paradox!

So, what's the solution?

The Bible says, *"Even if we feel guilty, God is greater than our feelings, and He knows everything"* (1 John 3:20 NLT). This verse can teach us how to manage our guilty feelings.

John reminds us to set our hearts on God's love. We free our minds by realizing that our feelings aren't facts, and therefore are not great decision-makers. We free our minds by recognizing God's voice over the voice of guilt and condemnation. God's voice does not produce guilt (Romans 8:1). His voice is one of assurance and comfort.

Choose to follow God's will for your life and refuse to let your feelings dictate how you should or should not respond. Let the

Word of God dictate your decisions, then set your mind to be a blessing—to make the choice that honors God.

If you break your boundaries (sin; give in to your flesh), repent— meaning, accept what you've done, and **sincerely** tell God that you're sorry and don't do it again.

First, we're often not sincere in our repentance; and second, we have not trusted God or even asked Him to help us stop the behavior. Ask the Holy Spirit to show you the source of your guilt. Guilt is rooted in low self-esteem and feelings of failure.

Finally ... remind, receive, recognize

Remind yourself that you are doing the best you can. Accept God's grace and know that you are where you are because of what God is trying to teach you, and until you learn the lesson, you need to be there. Ask Him what He's trying to show you. Remind yourself that a spirit of guilt will not motivate you to change and will only make you feel worse about yourself, which will lead you to eat or rebel against your health goals.

Receive God's grace and know that grace is not giving yourself permission to continue unhealthy habits. Grace is a gift from God to you.

Recognize that God is greater than your feelings of guilt. Recognize that feelings are not facts and are not reliable sources from which to make decisions.

My sister (and enlightened brother), it's time to cast out the spirit of guilt from your weight releasing program and your life. It is not from God. God convicts; He will never condemn you or make you feel guilty. Root out the spirit of guilt and start experiencing the joy, peace, and freedom that Christ died for us to experience, even in the midst of your short-comings, trials, missteps, and slip-ups.

Overcoming Guilt- Part Two - Living a Guilt-Free Life

"Even if we feel guilty, God is greater than our feelings, and He knows everything." (1 John 3:20 NLT)

I remember a friend once said to me, *"You feel guilty about everything."* Until then, I never realized how often I felt guilty. No matter what I did, I used to feel guilty about it. Years later, I realized that feeling guilty was my way of punishing myself for my actions. Unfortunately, this punishment never led to a change of behavior. It only left me feeling even worse about myself.

Do you suffer from always feeling guilty? Maybe you feel guilty that you ate more than you wanted; you missed your workout again; you missed your prayer time; or you did not do enough, give enough, try harder, or love more. Our feelings can plague us with so much guilt that often we go to bed every night feeling condemned and wake up the next morning feeling the same way.

Realize that just because you feel a certain way does not mean what we feel is true. We have to learn to separate our feelings from facts. There is very little place for guilt in the life of a believer. Feeling guilty is very destructive to your mind and really is nothing more than a subtle form of self-abuse or self-punishment. It makes us feel bad about ourselves or our actions, but it rarely inspires us to change our behavior or take action, so it really serves no purpose. In fact, it actually will hinder your progress instead of help it.

Remember this . . . **Satan condemns; The Holy Spirit convicts**. Feeling guilty can sometimes feel like a noble thing to do to motivate us to action, but notice the root of guilt—it is not from God, and therefore should be dismissed.

"Therefore, there is now no condemnation for those who are in Christ Jesus." (Romans 8:1)

What we want to feel is conviction. When the Holy Spirit corrects or convicts us, He will show us what we did wrong and show us how to correct it. He won't keep reminding you of your mistakes day-in and day-out, and have you continually feeling bad about what you did. He will expect you to move on once you have repented and taken responsibility for your actions.

In the scripture above, John offers an escape from this torture chamber of our minds. He reminds us to set our hearts on God's love when we feel guilt-ridden. We free our minds from feelings of guilt by realizing that our feelings aren't facts, and therefore are not great decision-makers. We free our minds by recognizing God's voice of correction and conviction over the enemy's voice of guilt and condemnation. God's voice will never make us feel guilty, no matter what we've done. His voice is one of assurance and comfort.

So, whether you ate more than you wanted, you yelled harshly at your child, you overspent on your budget, or you missed yet another workout, refuse to be plagued by feelings of guilt and condemnation. Spend time with God, repent of your actions, and move on. There is no benefit to wallowing in guilt.

Choose to follow God's will for your life, and refuse to let your guilty feelings dictate how you should or should not respond. Let the Word of God dictate your decisions, then set your mind to be a blessing to make right choices that honor God.

Prayer:

Dear Lord, thank You that You are so much greater than my feelings!! I've been dragged around by them into all kinds of situations that have left me full of shame and guilt. In many ways, God, I have made my feelings my lord and let them rule over me in the place that You belong as my only authority. I've done what I hate so many times because of my feelings—usually trying to avoid the ones that feel awful, but sometimes just to enjoy the ones that feel great. Please forgive me, Lord!

Today, I am trusting in Your unconditional love and in the knowledge that You are so much greater than my feelings! Help me please to trust in You when I start to feel tempted to let my feelings be my boss. Reassure me in my hour (or split second!) of need that Your ways are so much greater than mine, and that includes my feelings.

Give me the patience to pause before acting on my feelings, allowing them to just be. My desire is to grow so close to You and to know You so intimately and closely, sweet Lord! Instead of stuffing down and burying them, Lord, I will trust You with my feelings and experience the freedom, peace, and joy that Your compassion brings! You are truly awesome, God! In Jesus' name. Amen!

~ Geri Parisella

Overcoming Your Fear of Failure

Almost every day I hear from someone who says they are afraid of failing again.

It's understandable to get frustrated on the journey, but there are many things you can do to help you overcome your fear of failing so you can start succeeding at achieving your goal of achieving and maintaining healthy weight.

Fear of failure has negative consequences on your success. People who have a fear of failure are so worried about failing, that they often stop trying or give up just before they're about to reach their goal.

They don't realize that failing is what creates the steppingstones for our greatest success.

We would never question that in order for a piano player to excel in his craft, it would require many hours of practice. The same goes for any athlete or artist. Yet, we often don't realize that the same rules apply to our weight loss journey.

It's the principle of 'failing forward' otherwise known as 'practice', and it's necessary in order to lose weight and transform your habits.

Think about a baby learning to walk. You would never call them a failure every time they fell down, would you? What about a world-class figure skater preparing for the Olympics? The same principle applies to losing weight.

Everything you've learned in life has come through failing at first and then learning from your mistakes.

Unfortunately, many of us let our fear of failing keep us from achieving our goals. When you don't succeed, you say, "I'm a failure," rather than "I failed at this and now it's time to course-correct". The thought of failure can be debilitating and may be preventing you from taking action.

Here are some ways that your fear of failure can keep you from achieving your weight loss goals:

- You're afraid to start a diet because you don't think that you will be able to succeed.
- You hold on to 'fat-clothes' in case you gain the weight back.
- You may spend a lot of time researching health- and fitness-related materials but never take action.
- You may make a lot of excuses about why you can't lose weight, when deep down inside it's really fear.

How to overcome your fear of failure

See Every Set-Back as a Set-up for a Comeback!

"I do not consider myself yet to have taken hold of it. But one thing I do: Forgetting what is behind and straining toward what is ahead." (Philippians 3:13)

See failure as a learning opportunity—nothing more, nothing less. It does not mean you're a failure and it does not mean that you will fail again in the future, if you choose to see the lesson in every failure.

Sometimes God needs us to understand failure before He can bring about success with us. Just imagine what would happen if you woke up tomorrow at your ideal weight. Would you change your habits? Would you learn how to take care of yourself?

Would you learn how to love yourself, trust God, or learn patient endurance?

So, if you don't release weight one week (or two or three), instead of quitting use it as an opportunity to learn what you need to adjust for the coming week. Did you consume too much sodium? Did you eat too much? Did you eat too late at night? Were you too busy to exercise? If so, how can you adjust your schedule? Don't just say, 'Oh well, there's always next week.'Commit to doing better.

Seek Forgiveness

> "Seeing their faith, Jesus said to the paralytic, 'Take courage, son; your sins are forgiven.'" (Matthew 9:2 NASB 1995)

Every time you backslide, seek forgiveness for dishonoring your body and let God know your desire to get healthy. Our guilt and condemnation can often weigh us down and make us feel like a failure.

Isn't it interesting that when Jesus healed the paralyzed man, He did not comment on his ability to walk? His comment to him was, "...your sins are forgiven." Jesus recognized the man's spiritual health was so important, and that's the greater gift that Jesus gave the man. In faith, we must seek forgiveness for when we stumble. This will positively restore our body, soul, and spirit.

Live in Hope

> "Be strong and let your heart take courage, all you who hope in the LORD." (Psalms 31:24 ESV)

It can be so easy to feel like a failure when you want to do one thing but keep doing the exact opposite!

Despite our frustration, we must remain hopeful.

The Bible has so much to say about hope (Romans 8:24, 1 Corinthians 13:13, Hebrews 11:1). Hope is confidence and certainty that God will fulfill every promise He has made. Hope is confident assurance.

2 Corinthians 3:12 teaches us that our relationship with Christ gives us such confidence that we can be very bold, which means we can be confident in His power when we call on Him to help us. How would you rate your level of hope? To stop your fear of failure from derailing your weight loss efforts, take some time and study scriptures on hope (Hebrews 11:1-2; Corinthians 3:7-18).

Practice Progress, not Perfection

Too often we get so hung up on doing things just right that we miss all the little things that are making a big difference. We're only focused on the number on the scale and don't realize how much we're changing on the inside. We struggle with habits because we're focused on the outcome. Then we fall short of our expectations and get disappointed. Learning to keep practicing will require a shift in perspective. On your health journey, as well as other areas of your life, shift your focus to the process instead of being attached to the outcome.

In Philippians, Paul writes to the Philippian church and teaches them about the power of practice. He says, *"What you have learned and received and heard and seen in me—practice these things, and the God of peace will be with you."* (ESV)

Ask yourself, "What is truly keeping me from achieving my weight loss goals?" You might be surprised that it's a fear of failure. If so, let God know your fears and ask Him for guidance.

The Secret to Getting and Staying Out of Weight Loss Overwhelmedness

If you struggle with your weight, there's a high probability that you're often in a state of overwhelmedness.

Overwhelmedness comes from a feeling of 'too much', which, put another way, are also feelings of 'not enough' on your part—you don't have enough time, talent, skills, etc. to do what you need to do.

When you can discover how to 'get out of and stay out of overwhelmedness', many other areas of your life will start to fall into place—especially your weight.

- When you're overwhelmed, it's almost impossible to focus because your mind is always overrun with too many thoughts that keep you from experiencing God's peace and rest.

- When you're overwhelmed, you feel like you need to control everyone and everything. This gives you a false sense of control, because you're actually out of control.

- When you're overwhelmed you don't make good decisions, because you're unable to focus on what's really important, it's hard to 'see the forest for the trees.'

- When you're overwhelmed, you're always jumping from thing to thing—looking for the quickest and easiest solution instead of taking the time to focus on what matters most.

- When you're overwhelmed, you look for ways to stop the insanity that is your life, so you use things like food, drugs, shopping, TV, or other things to distract you.

- When you're overwhelmed, God's voice gets drowned out among all the dozens of to-dos, schedules, and plans.

Getting Out of Overwhelmedness

How do you stop without feeling like your life will come crashing down?

1. See Overwhelmedness as a Spirit.

Personify it as an enemy created (by self) to keep you from moving towards your purpose. When you can see it from this perspective, you'll recognize that it's not part of who you are and can be eliminated from your life.

2. Recognize That It's a Form of Procrastination

Being overwhelmed is the perfect scapegoat for rationalizing why you can't do the things you want to do.

How can you possibly exercise when you have so much to do? How can you spend time with God when people are relying on you and you 'need to' get this job done? The question to ask yourself is, 'What are you really afraid of?' If you were not doing all of the things that are keeping you busy, what would you really be doing? Yeah, that thing—that's what you're hiding from.

3. Move From Doing to Being

Overwhelmed people are always looking for a way to fix things. "How do I?" is the constant question. "How do I solve this? How do I fix this? How do I help them? How do I change?" This constant search for the answer is what keeps you overwhelmed. Stop it! Instead of asking, "How do I?", take a deep breath and ask God what He wants you to learn in this situation. Be someone led by the spirit of God instead of always trying to figure things out. God calls us to '**be** holy' (1 Peter 1:6 (emphasis added)). Being does not involve a three-step plan or a checklist. It's actually the opposite. Freedom from overwhelmedness comes when you stop running around like a chicken with your head cut off and stand still before God and let Him direct your path. Right where you are right now, stop for a second and take a deep breath and invite the Holy Spirit into your life. Stop from all your worry and work and just be in His presence. (Psalms 40:10).

Staying Out of Overwhelmedness

Okay... so that was one breath! What's next, you might be wondering.

Staying out of overwhelmedness will require you to learn some new habits, but before you get ready to write down the secret and get busy doing it, recognize that it ain't that kind of secret. Staying out of overwhelmedness requires the work of the Holy Spirit working in you. It's not something you muster up in your own strength. That's what got you in this situation in the first place!

- You manage your overwhelmedness one day at a time; one action at a time; one decision at a time with God as your strength.

- Wake up and give your day to God—ask Him to lead you and guide you throughout the day.

- As you move from activity to activity, are you in a rush or are you taking God with you?

- Are you inviting God into the details of your life?

- Pray before making decisions, before answering requests, and before taking on new projects.

- Lay your desire to be healthy at His feet and ask Him to show you how to do it.

As you begin to entrust everything over to Him, He will begin to show you the patterns that keep you overwhelmed (over-giving, over-thinking, over-working, over-pleasing). He will show you what you're really afraid of at the right time, and this will happen with ease! Not that it will be easy, but it will not feel forced. It won't feel like another thing on your list, and you won't feel deprived or robbed of fun. You will be able to let go effortlessly and easily when God is in control.

Nice Girls Finish Fat: Is your People-Pleasing Keeping You Unhealthy and Overweight?

As a Christian weight loss coach and personal trainer, one of the behavioral patterns I often come across in people that keep them overweight is the 'People Pleaser' mentality.

People-pleasers are always apologizing, they are afraid of what other people would think, they feel that they're not good enough. They say yes when they often want to say no or they feel bad when they do say no. They excessively worry a lot, they often live to serve others, they often strive for perfection, and they take what people say about them very personally. Does this sound like you?

If so, hang tight, because starting today you can begin to change this pattern.

It seems absurd that people-pleasing can be tied to weight issues, but over the years of working with people, here are some of the connections I've made and learned.

How people-pleasing makes and keeps you overweight

1. Since people-pleasers put others first, they will eat foods they don't want to, to not 'offend' others. While we all do this on rare occasions, people-pleasers can make this routine. I have clients who eat high-fat and calorie-loaded dinners their husbands cook every night because they don't want to offend them.

2. At the root of people-pleasing is a fear of failure and fear of success. Fear of failure is rooted in feelings of inadequacy, and fear of success is rooted in feelings of overwhelmedness and rejection. People-pleasers can become so concerned with what people will think of them that they will subconsciously sabotage their weight loss goals for fear of judgment from themselves or from other people.

3. If you've spent most of your life being a people-pleaser, then you've become emotionally addicted to the need for people to validate you. And when you don't get it, you will eat to stuff the feelings of emptiness you feel or, conversely, you will eat to seek the reward that you did not get externally. Subconsciously you feel that if no one is going to make you feel better, then you might as well make yourself feel better with food. The problem is that this addiction, like all others, is insatiable.

> *"Am I now trying to win the approval of human beings, or of God? Or am I trying to please people? If I were still trying to please people, I would not be a servant of Christ."*
> (Galatians 1:10)

So now that you understand this, what do you do?

Although it's too much to go through in this article, here is a starting point to help you begin to change:

Step 1: Get to the Root

Through prayer ask God to show you what is at the root of your people-pleasing. In the course we go through guided exercises to help you get there.

Step 2: Let Go

Although easier said than done, you will learn to:

- let go of your story
- let go of the people who want you to please them
- let go of your need to be liked
- let go of your need to be needed
- let go of your need for approval
- let go of the fears that keep you stuck
- let go of the unproductive language that you've been using to keep you stuck in your story

When you learn to let go, you will begin to attract affirming people, situations, and events in your life that will begin to shape a new identity for you; an identity that is based on Christ and not on what man thinks.

Are You the Queen of Procrastination?

Are you always putting off your workouts or telling yourself you'll start tomorrow? You're not alone. Procrastination is a serious barrier that stops us from reaching our goals.

We can look to the New Testament to see the consequences of procrastination (Luke 9:59-62, Luke 14:15-24).

In the parable of the Great Feast in Luke 14: 15-24, many people turned down the invitation to the banquet (God's blessings) because the timing was inconvenient. Unfortunately, they all deferred action and missed out on a wonderful opportunity because of their procrastination.

In the Message Bible, Jesus' responses to the men who wanted to put off following Him was this: "Jesus said, 'No procrastination. No backward looks. You can't put God's kingdom off till tomorrow. Seize the day'." (Luke 9:62)

How about you? Jesus may also be calling us to stop procrastinating.

Do you also keep putting off your health program and/or weight releasing program?

If you need help, here are some reasons we procrastinate and some practical steps you can take to root out this debilitating habit.

Feeling overwhelmed can lead to procrastination

Have you ever had so much to do that you end up spending the evening on the couch, watching Netflix? It's common. When your mind has too much going on, it basically goes into shut-down mode.

Solution? Do a brain dump. Write out on paper everything that is consuming your thoughts. Once it's out on paper, your mind will be more clear to process what it needs to get done. Then you can begin to prioritize what's most important.

Feeling lazy from poor lifestyle choices can lead to procrastination

It's a Catch 22—the more you move and eat healthy foods, the more energy you'll have and the less you'll procrastinate. Too often, we feel so sluggish that the thought of moving or doing anything feels impossible.

Solution? Start small. What healthy choices can you make today to kick those feelings of laziness? Select something you can do right now to boost your energy. Drink water? Go outside for some fresh air? Call a friend?

Feeling unmotivated can lead to procrastination

Without goals and dreams, it's hard to get (and stay motivated). When you're not living the life God has called you to live, you can feel discouragement and the lack of motivation to get moving. If you're not inspired by your fitness goals, then chances are you will not strive to accomplish them. What will really motivate you this year?

Solution? Take some time and understand what really moves and inspires you. What do you love doing? What brings you peace, joy, freedom? If you're not sure, spend time in prayer and ask the Holy Spirit to remind you what used to make you happy—taking up hiking, taking up a new sport, mountain climbing? Get busy planning how you're going to dream again and start living from those dreams!

Feeling undisciplined can lead to procrastination

Are you hit and miss with your workouts? Or maybe one week you planned all your meals for the week and the next week, you went right back to eating out? Frustrating, isn't it?

Solution? So, what do you do when you just don't feel like working out? First, understand that self-discipline is like a muscle. The more you use it, the stronger it becomes. So regardless of how you're feeling right now, ask yourself what small thing you can do to help strengthen your discipline muscle. There really is no easy answer. You've got to put in the time, but remember it's a process and change will take place little by little once you stay the course.

Fear can lead to procrastination

Sometimes, we're so afraid of failing that we never start. In our minds, it's easier to put things off instead of facing the possibility that we might not be successful.

Solution? Get to the root of what fears are holding you back. Whether it's fear of failure or some other fear that may be stopping you, know that all fears are an opportunity to allow God to fulfill an unmet core need in your life. It could be a need for love, acceptance, security, or fulfillment. Take a moment and write out what the fear is and turn it into a prayer. For example, if you're afraid of failing again pray and ask God for fulfillment and success in Him and through Him. All of our fears can be turned into opportunities for prayer.

You might find yourself procrastinating because of one, or even several, of the reasons listed above. Start with one and begin today to take baby steps to stop procrastinating and start moving forward, trusting God as your strength.

Chapter Five

The Word on Weight Loss

What do Oprah and Samson Have in Common?

Have you ever noticed that being strong in one area of your life does not necessarily have a cross-over effect? You can be totally competent in one area of your life and be the complete opposite in another. This point became even more apparent to me as I was reading about the story of Samson in Judges 13-16.

The Lord endowed Samson with superhuman strength, and he used it against Israel's enemies and led the nation for twenty years. In one conflict, he killed one thousand Philistine men. He was powerful, undefeatable, and a leader, so what went wrong? Despite his strength, his flesh craved what he knew he should have avoided (Philistine women). His story reminded me of the cover of one of the tabloid magazines I saw as I was standing in line at the checkout counter. It said, 'Oprah 200 lbs—"How Could I Let this Happen Again."'

Many of us can identify with Oprah. You're on a roll, you're doing so well, it seems like you've finally kicked this weight thing (or other issue), and then, 'BAM!', you start again on that all too familiar slippery slope. The next thing you know, you've sabotaged yourself again. You feel like victory will never be yours.

Like Samson in the Bible, you would think that Oprah would be the least likely person to fail. Samson seemed to have everything going for him. He was dedicated to God from birth, possessed incredible strength, and had amazing parents.

Oprah has personal chefs, personal assistants, and personal trainers at her disposal 24 hours a day. If anyone should be able to keep weight off, it should be Oprah, right? Yet both of these 'giants' were not able to move past their appetites.

So, the question becomes, "What are we mere mortals to do?" If these powerhouses could not control their flesh, then what chance do we have?

And this is the point—**we don't stand a chance** against our appetites and sensual desires. We really are powerless to change ourselves. God wants us to draw our strength from Him in every area of our lives, especially in the area that seems impossible, like our weight.

We often deceive ourselves by believing that if only we could afford a personal trainer or if only we had the time to make the right foods, then we would lose weight. If only we had more time in our schedule or if only we had more motivation.

It's not about trying harder or doing more; it's about giving God full reign in our lives. With His guidance, an organized plan, and some accountability we can have success finally and forever!

Despite His strengths highlighted in the Bible, Samson played by his own rules. He violated many of God's laws, was controlled by his flesh, and confided in the wrong people. Can you see how you also may not be totally submitted to God?

It's never too late to start over. Learn from Samson (and Oprah) and submit your weight release to God. He is more than able to handle it. This principle of submitting to God is exactly what our 10-Day Challenge (10daysgodsway.com) is all about.

A Common Sense Weight Loss Approach from Scripture

Have you ever thought about the Bible as offering a common-sense approach to weight loss? Just like answers to every other challenge in life, it's in there.

We use the name *Weight Loss, God's Way* for our online program because I truly believe that a biblical approach to weight loss is the best route. We often feel we need a complex plan in order to have the greatest success. If it's simple we think it's not worth trying, but the Word is full of common-sense instructions for daily living. God wants us to "get it", and common sense is a gift He has given us to apply it.

That feeling in the pit of our stomach is common sense. It often gets ignored. It's like a warning light notifying us that we are ready to make a bad decision. More importantly, it's the Holy Spirit directing us to make the right choice.

It's time we not only listen to those promptings, but ask for more of the same. The Holy spirit can and will help us reach our health and weight loss goals if we only ask Him. We just have to be ready to take action when we hear His voice. Often, His voice comes through His written Word.

There are many scriptures that can lead us on our journey. Here are some principles we can apply today to make impact:

5 Common-Sense Principles

1. Common sense tells us to do first things first. We have a tendency to put off what's important. We know that we should

exercise, but other things continue to become more of a priority. They take our focus and our time.

What do you keep putting off? If it's exercise, do it first thing in the morning so nothing else gets in the way. Lay out your gym clothes at the end of the bed so they are there waiting for you in the morning. Take a small step towards making exercise a priority.

Proverbs 14:15 teaches us that wise people carefully consider their steps.

2. Common sense tells us to use the day wisely. Instead of taking the time to grocery shop for the right foods, plan our meals for the week, and carve out some time to go to the gym, we get side-tracked by surfing the internet, watching Netflix, or playing Candy Crush.

Plan out your health goals the day before and don't allow anything to sidetrack you. What time of the day do you have the most energy? Schedule and plan to work hardest during that time. Can you double batch some meals to save time? Wisdom teaches us that if we don't drink enough water we'll feel sluggish, so drink up! That will help you get the most out of your day.

Psalm 90:12 teaches us to number our days so we can gain wisdom on how to best spend our time.

3. Common sense tells us that if something is not working, then we should stop doing it, but we keep making the same mistakes over and over again, expecting different results.

We know that diets don't work, yet we can't seem to resist the urge and lure of trying the latest one. Each day, review what strategies worked and what didn't work and adjust accordingly.

Decide to not continue the same broken patterns that just aren't working.

James 1:5 teaches us that if we lack wisdom we should ask God. He will help us so that we don't keep making the same mistakes over and over again.

4. Common sense tells us to focus on what's important, but we tend to major on the minors. We can get caught up in things that don't matter and go a whole day without even giving God a thought or giving Him thanks for all He has blessed us with. Too often we frustrate ourselves looking for answers to problems, then go to Him when we have tried everything else and had it fail.

Asking God for His wisdom, peace, direction and even strength for making right choices should be part of our daily living. He wants to lead us. He wants a relationship with us. Every day He wants us to submit our weight-loss journey to Him. We cannot do this in our own strength.

If we are obsessed with weight loss, that is not of Him either. Ask God for a healthy balance and perspective. If we put Him first, everything else will fall in place and we will have peace.

Matthew 6:33 tells us to seek first God's kingdom and everything else will be added unto us.

5. Common sense tells us that hard work will pay off. Many of us want results, but we're just not willing to do the work it takes to achieve our goals. It's time to be honest with ourselves. It is going to take some discipline, sweat, and sacrifice to gain the victory. There is no easy way around it. Ask yourself if you are willing to do what it takes to get the results you want. Know it will be worth it if your answer is "yes."

Proverbs 14:23 teaches us that work brings profit, but mere talk leads to poverty.

God Is For You

God is not silent about how He wants us to live our lives. Let's continue to use the wisdom and common-sense principles that He has provided. Take action today to achieve your goals and know that His desire is for your success. 3 John 1:2 says, *"Beloved, I pray that in all respects you may prosper and be in good health, just as your soul prospers."* (NASB) **Know it, believe it, and trust Him.**

A Weight Loss Lesson from Joshua: How Long Will You Wait?

Here's the scene:

Moses had died and Joshua was now in charge. He had been leading the Israelites when he noticed that they had yet to take possession of what was theirs. And so, he asked, "How long will you wait before you begin to take possession of the land that the Lord, the God of your ancestors, has given you?"

I can imagine how some of the Israelites reacted. "What does he mean, how long will we wait? We've been circling this mountain for 40 years and we can finally see the promised land. We made it." Though they had finally made it around that mountain, they still had something in them that was preventing them from taking what was theirs. I mean, God had promised them this land and there it was, and they still hadn't taken hold of it. Why???

Sometimes in our weight loss journey, we forget that good health is our inheritance. It is what God has had for us from the beginning. And through this journey, we can become like the Israelites.

We can circle around the same mountains or habits for 40 years or more. Still struggling with meal prepping, still struggling with sugar consumption, still struggling with binge-eating, and finally, one day, we look up and we see the promised land.

We may have lost all but 5 pounds of our goal weight, or we may be down to drinking just one soda a week, and we can literally see the promise of God. Yet, we don't go in and finish it off.

We don't go in and take full claim of what's ours. We become satisfied with living right outside our promise. We're happy with only losing 3/4 of the weight we wanted to lose. We're satisfied with drinking one soda a week. We walk around with the notion of, "Hey, it's better than what it was three months ago, right???"

Here's the thing: When we set a goal to get to good health, we should NEVER SETTLE for almost attaining it. We must take this scripture and see it as it truly is, and ask ourselves how long are we going to wait before we truly go in and take action concerning our health?

If you notice in the scripture, Joshua implied that the Israelites had to take action themselves to claim the land. It wasn't just handed over to them. Joshua didn't go and divide it up for them. They had to go in and take action to claim what was theirs.

Moral of the story: My dear friends, I ask each of you, how long will it be until you take possession of what God has for you?

I know for myself, I am tired of sitting outside the promised land looking in. Being near it no longer satisfies me. I want ALL that God promises me, and I will go in and take claim of what is mine!

We provide so many tools to help you to start AND finish this journey once and for all. I implore you to gather your strength in the Lord and take possession of your health.

Get Out of the Boat! Weight Loss Lessons from the Apostle Peter

As Christians, we should view weight loss as a faith walk. A call to live out the scriptures that teach us to rely on our Heavenly Father for our strength, sustenance, and satisfaction. It's a lesson about testing in times of trials, submission in times of willful disobedience, and trust in times of anxiety and disappointment.

What makes Christian weight loss different is that it's not about how sexy we look in our jeans, or how toned and sculpted we can get. There is nothing wrong with having these goals, but if that is your only motivation for getting healthier then it will be a long journey of deprivation with little reward at the end.

We all know that the lure of obtaining the ideal body is very tempting, and the majority of women will be seduced by its pull, but remember that we are called to be so much more. Despite what society would have us believe, we are so much more than our bodies, and our self-worth is not determined by our measurements.

The story of Peter came to my mind this week. It goes like this ...

> *"Immediately Jesus made the disciples get into the boat and go on ahead of him to the other side, while he dismissed the crowd. After he had dismissed them, he went up on a mountainside by himself to pray. Later that night, he was there alone, and the boat was already a considerable*

distance from land, buffeted by the waves because the wind was against it.

Shortly before dawn Jesus went out to them, walking on the lake. When the disciples saw him walking on the lake, they were terrified. "It's a ghost," they said, and cried out in fear.

But Jesus immediately said to them: "Take courage! It is I. Don't be afraid."

"Lord, if it's you," Peter replied, "tell me to come to you on the water."

"Come," he said.

Then Peter got down out of the boat, walked on the water and came toward Jesus. But when he saw the wind, he was afraid and, beginning to sink, cried out, "Lord, save me!"

Immediately Jesus reached out his hand and caught him. "You of little faith," he said, "why did you doubt?"

And when they climbed into the boat, the wind died down. Then those who were in the boat worshiped him, saying, 'Truly you are the Son of God.'" (Matthew 14:22-33)

Does Peter's scenario seem familiar to you?

How many times has God spoken to you? Like Peter, you hear Him, you see Him working in your life and are strengthened to do what seems impossible. You're eating healthy, making time to be active, spending time in His Word, saying 'no' to all the distractions. You're doing it! You're actually doing it!

Then it happens ... the phone call; the coworkers' harsh words; your husband's rejecting tone—the familiar feelings of insignificance. Whatever it is, that is your 'wind' that makes you feel like that scared little girl who needs food for comfort.

That's the 'wind' that blows through your mind and temporarily makes you forget that with Christ all things are possible. It's the same familiar 'wind' that continually blows through your mind and causes you to sink.

If only we could remember that the hunger pangs, the anxiety, and the negative feelings will pass. If only we could remember that the wind will die down once the fear subsides.

Here are three lessons that you can learn about your health and weight loss journey from the story of Peter walking on water:

1. To walk on water will take faith, not fear.

> *"Come." So Peter got out of the boat and walked on the water and came to Jesus. But when he saw the wind, he was afraid, and beginning to sink he cried out, "Lord, save me." Jesus immediately reached out his hand and took hold of him, saying to him, "O you of little faith, why did you doubt?"* (Matthew 14:29–32 ESV)

We hear it all the time. 'Have faith', 'Just have faith', but how can we have faith when we may have grown up always feeling fearful? Peter and the disciples just finished witnessing Jesus feeding 5,000 men with five loaves and two fishes (Matt. 14:18). How could they lose their faith so quickly?

The Bible teaches us to keep our eyes fixed on Jesus (Heb. 12:2). When we're not thinking, it's so easy to forget that our strength comes from Christ and Christ alone.

Peter was actually walking on water! He had faith enough to believe he could do it. So, what happened?

"But when he saw the wind, he was afraid and, beginning to sink, cried out, "Lord, save me!" (Matt. 14:30). He quickly moved from faith to fear. He took his eyes off Jesus and let his fear take control. Isn't that just how we do it? One minute we're feeling safe and secure in our Father's presence, and in the blink of an eye fear creeps in and we're blinded by it.

I'm learning that faith is a minute-by-minute decision, not something that you get and it stays with you forever. Fear will come, but as soon as it does remember to call out to Jesus, and He will reach out His hand to rescue you. Before you reach for the potato chips, before you feel like you're going to die if you don't eat something, call out to Jesus as Peter did. He will help you when you can't help yourself.

2. If you want to walk on water, you've got to get out of the boat.

"...made them get into the boat and go before him to the other side" (Matt 14:22).

The journey that we are called to walk will not be easy, but it is necessary to strengthen us. Notice that it was Jesus who sent the disciples out late **and** on a stormy night. He could have sent them in the middle of the day when the weather was nice and calm. They would not have had any need to fear and they certainly would not have had a need to trust in Jesus. That's just like us. When things are going well, we often forget that we are weak and fearful. Without our health and weight challenges, we would have no need to call out for help. Like the disciples, it's in the dark stormy times when we can't see our way when we call out to Him, and that's when He always shows up. See your weight from a different perspective; see it as a 'check engine' light in your car telling you that you are in need of the Savior.

If you feel like you're never going to lose the weight, remember that's the time to stretch out your hand like Peter and let the Holy Spirit remind you to take courage and not be afraid (v. 27). Like Peter, Jesus will also reach out His hand to us when we are afraid.

3. If you fall, it's not fatal.

Peter's story did not end with his sinking. This story ends with a beautiful, comforting ending of Jesus reaching out His hand and catching him (v. 31). But wait, the story gets even better! Fast forward a few years later and we read that Peter grew to become one of the leading figures in the church. In 1 Peter 7-9, he teaches us that:

> *"These have come so that the proven genuineness of your faith—of greater worth than gold, which perishes even though refined by fire—may result in praise, glory and honor when Jesus Christ is revealed. Though you have not seen him, you love him; and even though you do not see him now, you believe in him and are filled with an inexpressible and glorious joy, for you are receiving the end result of your faith, the salvation of your souls."*

What a testimony coming from someone who was just feet away from Jesus and was still afraid. His testing and trials strengthened his faith as nothing else could. The boat experience was not tragic; in fact, it was a steppingstone to greater things. He needed to go through that experience to strengthen his faith and his relationship with Christ.

This can also be your testimony on your weight loss journey. Like Peter, let's use our trials to help us overcome our fears as we learn to trust in our Heavenly Father to meet our every need.

Weight Loss Lessons from the Book of Daniel

Trying to lose weight? Consistency and discipline are important keys to helping you reach your goal. Learn from the story of Daniel how focus, consistency, and discipline are crucial to reaching your goals.

It still amazes me how easy it is to get off track with your health goals. I was on a great roll recording my food. I was consistently using myfitnesspal.com and finally got serious about keeping my 'carbs' in check (that's my 'weakness'). Then I went to Antigua for four days last week, where the internet was not so great, and that's all it took for me to 'fall off the wagon.' Although I started tracking again, I still have not gotten back into doing it consistently.

Does this ever happen to you? Maybe food tracking is not your thing. Maybe it's developing consistency with your exercise program, or not eating after a certain hour. You're going along great, then 'life' throws you a curve ball. Maybe it's a death in the family, a vacation, or you get sick, but the next thing you know what seemed like a sure thing feels like a distant memory. It can be very frustrating, to say the least.

There's a very short but powerful sentence in the book of Daniel that offers up some great advice and perspective on how to maintain your focus when life throws you a curveball. Most of us would never pick up on this scripture, but once you go deeper, you'll see how powerful it is:

And Daniel continued even to the first year of King Cyrus.
(Daniel 1:21 NKJV)

And Daniel continued... Daniel was one of the first Jewish captives taken into Babylon, and he lived to see the end of their captivity. He lived to see the promises of Isaiah and Jeremiah fulfilled, which spoke about the exiles returning to their home in Jerusalem in the first year of King Cyrus, 70 years after his captivity.

Daniel continued... He maintained his religion, customs, and even his diet for 70 years in a foreign land.

Daniel continued... He obeyed all of God's laws, made up his mind not to defile himself despite all the pressures around him to conform and compromise.

How did Daniel survive all those years in a foreign land? He prayed for God's help and maintained his integrity.

We can learn so much from Daniel. When we experience change we can feel so lost, but like Daniel we can pray for God's help each and every day and God will help us in our times of need.

Like Daniel, purpose in your heart to never quit because you know how difficult it is to restart. The best way to maintain momentum is to never stop. It may be difficult for you to start, but once you do you will gain momentum that will propel you to keep going. The next time you think of quitting or throwing in the towel, remember all of the wonderful momentum you've already gained and how much you will regret your decision to quit.

Let's try to model our health like Daniel did and **continue,** regardless of the circumstances.

What the Story of the Widow's Mite Can Teach Us About Getting in Shape

Want to exercise, but can't seem to make the time?

Or maybe you can't justify the expense and effort to eat healthier foods, then make the time to prepare them?

For many of us we truly desire to be in better health, but when the rubber meets the road it's hard to do what it actually takes to see the results we want.

There's a powerful story in the Bible that can teach us about commitment to our health, and how I believe God wants us to live in this area of our lives. It's the story of the widow's mite in Mark 12:41-44.

> "Jesus sat down opposite the place where the offerings were put and watched the crowd putting their money into the temple treasury. Many rich people threw in large amounts. But a poor widow came and put in two very small copper coins, worth only a few cents.
>
> Calling his disciples to him, Jesus said, 'Truly I tell you, this poor widow has put more into the treasury than all the others. They all gave out of their wealth; but she, out of her poverty, put in everything—all she had to live on.'"

So, what does this have to do with my health, you may be asking?

As Christians, we know that God owns everything and has called us to steward them—our finances, our gifts, our health, they all belong to Him. But He has called us to be representatives of it all—stewarding it in a way that is responsible.

In the same way, Scripture tells us that our bodies are not our own, they belong to God, and we have a responsibility to care for them.

> *"You are not your own, for you were bought with a price. So glorify God in your body."* (1 Corinthians 6:19-20 ESV)

So, let's go back to the widow's mite.

Jesus' principle here teaches us a few things about how God wants us to steward everything in our possession.

1. Steward with trust

Whether it's 10 pounds, 100 pounds, or 300 pounds we want to release, God wants us to trust HIM to meet all our needs just like the widow trusted by giving all she had. There was no Plan B for her and there was no opportunity to take matters into her own hands if things did not work out as she hoped. She did not keep one mite and give the other—she gave it all. She trusted God one hundred percent!

Can you say the same for you on your health journey? Are you giving all you have, or are you holding back? Do you really trust God to help you achieve a healthy weight, or do you keep taking matters into your own hands? Do you keep jumping from diet to diet and program to program, or are you submitting this journey to Him and listening to how He is leading and guiding you? Don't be afraid to ask yourself these questions.

We know that Jesus was pleased with her offering because she gave all she had. She did not hold back. And we can believe that

He will also be pleased with us when we offer our bodies as a living sacrifice to him.

2. Steward with the right spirit

In the story of the widow's mite, we learn that the spirit of giving, or of anything else, determines the value of the gift more than the amount. Her two mites were of more value than all those who gave out of abundance.

God does not call us to do anything begrudgingly or, conversely, from a place of vanity like the other rich givers. He calls us to glorify Him in our body. He calls us to give from a place of sacrifice and worship.

So, ask yourself, when you think about exercise and healthy eating what is your predominant thought? Too hard? Too painful? It's deprivation? No time? Is it to weigh a certain number on the scale or to have the perfect body? The fact of the matter is that the manner in which you portray healthy habits in your mind will also determine your level of success or failure.

If you envision healthy habits as painful or as a means to fix other problems in your life, you won't stick with them very long. If you envision them as a form of worship or sacrifice to God—a way to glorify God in your body, a long-term blessing in your life—you will be more likely to stick with them, even when the going gets tough.

"Therefore, I urge you, brothers and sisters, in view of God's mercy, to offer your bodies as a living sacrifice, holy and pleasing to God—this is your true and proper worship."
(Romans 12:1)

3. Steward with the right thinking

The widow gave from where she was at. She gave what she had. She did not wait until her circumstances changed before she gave. She opposed the faulty mindset that says, *"I'll give when I have more."*

Too often we say, "I'll start my exercise program when I have more time, when I have more money, when my life finally settles down." The problem with this thinking is that it's always in the future and we keep putting it off. The next thing you know, ten years have passed, and we wonder where the time went and where all the excess weight came from. It also puts you in the driver's seat and does not allow you to rely on God to meet your needs.

There will never be a perfect time to start, so if this is your mindset then it's time to change. Today is a good day to start, regardless of how much time or how much money you have. You can always do something. And you can be confident that God will bless those small steps. Whatever we give sacrificially to God, we can be assured that He sees it and is pleased, just as He was with the widow.

For today, reflect on your stewardship of your body. Where do you need to make some adjustments? Check your trust, your spirit, and your thinking. Place your trust in God and ask Him to guide you towards a lifestyle of worship and sacrifice. Ask Him to help you become more like the widow. Just start from where you are right now.

Your Comfort or Your Calling—A Weight Loss Lesson from the Story of Esther

Many of us never reach our full potential. It's true whether it's fulfilling our calling, doing great things for God, or even being as healthy as we could be. Let's face it, if being healthy was easy then it would be a daily habit for us each day. The fitness industry would not be a billion-dollar industry, and our medical bills would be a lot lower. Success at anything takes hard work, discipline, consistency, and determination. We owe it to ourselves to stay the course and live a healthy life that we were designed to live.

Having said that, I hate to admit it, but comfort is one of my highest priorities in life. When I think of comfort, I think of a nice, warm, cozy bed, my slippers that look like oven mitts, and my favorite purple throw on the couch. Living comfortably also means not constantly under stress or pressure, not worrying about where my next meal is coming from or where I'm going to sleep.

However, there is also a downside of being comfortable. It means never stepping out of your comfort zone, never taking risks, never challenging myself, never sacrificing, and not doing things that are too onerous or difficult. It can be a big factor in what can keep you from reaching your full potential. I dislike this aspect of myself because it keeps me from learning new things, experiencing new opportunities, and growing.

Based on our personality, some of us are more adventurous than others. But regardless of where we are on the spectrum, we must not let our comfort get in the way of our calling. God led me to the story of Esther to teach me about the importance of getting uncomfortable in order to fulfill my calling.

The story of Esther is about a young Jewish orphan girl selected for the king's harem, who through a series of circumstances, miraculously becomes the Queen of Persia. Although God is not mentioned in the entire story, it demonstrates God's love and sovereignty when we step out boldly to do what seems difficult, challenging, or downright impossible.

I came upon two (what I consider) pivotal passages in the story;

> *"For if you remain silent at this time, relief and deliverance for the Jews will arise from another place, but you and your father's family will perish. And who knows but that you have come to your royal position for such a time as this? . . . and,*
> *"And if I perish, I perish."* (Esther 4:14,16)

After studying these two passages, I thought to myself, what if Ester did not step out of the familiar to the unfamiliar? What if she did not obey the calling that God had placed on her life? What if she was not willing to do what her uncle had asked her to do? What if she did not step out of her comfort zone and decide to risk it all? As I asked myself these questions, I could hear God asking me, *"Cathy, do you want to be comfortable all of your life or do you want to fulfill your calling?"*

My honest answer to Him was and is "both." I don't want one in exclusion of the other, and I don't think that God wants me to live an 'uncomfortable' life. But He showed me that there are times when I have to step out of my comfort zone. There are times when we have to do what it takes to promote change, to look outside ourselves and do things that are bigger than we ever thought we were capable of, and there are times where we have to take risks. Fortunately, it's usually for a season and is usually followed by a harvest (Ecc 3:1, Psalm 1:3). Sometimes we have to do what is difficult regardless of whether we feel like it or not.

As you read my testimony, I challenge you to ask yourself the same question about your health. Are you willing to do the uncomfortable tasks and actions? Are you willing to push through when you don't feel like it and when you are out of your comfort zone? Are you willing to wake up a bit earlier, turn off the TV and go for a walk instead, choose not to eat more than you know you should, and spend more time in prayer?

If your answer is a resounding "yes" like mine was, then get back on your horse and let's continue on this journey together. Keep submitting your health, your body, and your weight to God and let Him ease your burdens. That's His promise to you and to me.

I recommit to be led by my calling and not by my comfort level. Will you join me?

What to Do When You've Hit a Plateau: Psalms 23

In the weightlossgodsway.com program, we're in a 21-day Bible study called, "Messy in the Middle." It's helping those of us who feel like we're 'stuck' to allow God to bring us to the other side with grace and peace.

As we understand the process, we've come to understand that all weight loss journeys have a beginning, a middle, and an end.

Typically, when we begin a program, we're excited. Thankfully, we've temporarily forgotten our past attempts and are filled with optimism for what is to come. We believe that maybe this time it will be different.

The end of our journey is so rewarding! We've put in the time, we've paid the price, and our results reflect our sacrifice. We feel accomplished and victorious.

But it's the period in the middle of our weight loss journey that's the most challenging. It's the period in the middle where our willpower, enthusiasm, and motivation have worn off.

It's the period in the middle where the novelty of the adrenaline rush that often accompanies the newness of a task or project wears off. Where the excitement of the commitment we made at the start comes face to face with the reality of the work involved.

As we studied Psalms 23:4 during one of our "Seek Him Saturday" calls, we found great comfort in understanding that God is with us during the 'messy middles' of our journey. As we studied the Valley of the Shadow of Death, we learned that it is a real place. Check this out!!

"There is a valley of the shadow of death in the Holy Land. It is south of the Jericho Road leading from Jerusalem to the Dead Sea and is a narrow defile through the mountain range. Climatic and grazing conditions make it necessary for the sheep to be moved through this valley for seasonal feeding. "The valley is four and a half miles long. Its sidewalls are over 1500 feet high in places and it is only 10 or 12 feet wide at the bottom. Travel through the valley is dangerous, because its floor, badly eroded by cloudbursts, has deep gullies. Actual footing on solid rock is so narrow in places that a sheep cannot turn around, and it is an unwritten law of shepherds that flocks must go up the valley in the morning hours and down towards the eventide, lest flocks meet in the defile. Mules have not been able to make the trip for centuries, but sheep and goat herders from earliest Old Testament days have maintained a passage for their stock.

"About halfway through the valley, the walk crosses from one side to the other at a place where the path is cut in two by an eight-foot gully. One section of the path is about 18 inches higher than the other; the sheep must jump across it. The shepherd stands at this break and coaxes or forces the sheep to make the leap. If the sheep slips and lands in the gully, the shepherd's staff is brought into play. The old-style crook is encircled around a large sheep's neck or a small sheep's chest, and it is lifted to safety. If a more modern narrow crook is used, the sheep is caught about the hoofs and lifted up to the walk.

"Many wild dogs lurk in the shadows of the valley, looking for prey. After a band of sheep has entered the defile, the leader may come upon such a dog. Unable to retreat, the leader baas a warning. The shepherd, skilled in throwing his rod, hurls it

at the dog and knocks it into the washed-out gully where it is easily killed. Thus the sheep have learned to fear no evil, even in the valley of the shadow of death, for their master is there to aid them and protect them from harm."

Taken from an article by James K. Wallace, who quotes the words of Ferando D'Alphonso, an experienced shepherd.

If you're also moving through a messy middle, take comfort that our Good Shepherd is with us in the midst of our trials, leading us and protecting us. We're not alone, and we will make it to the other side if we persevere, trusting God to get us safely to the other side.

Are you going through a valley at the moment? What comfort, encouragement, and strength can you take from these verses?

I pray that you were blessed by this compilation of my blog posts over the last 15 years. My philosophies and my approach may have changed over the years, but the one thing that will always remain is God's Word and its impact on our health and every area of our lives if we allow it. Commit to keep on surrendering your health journey to God, commit to spending time in His Word, and commit to doing what He says to do and the battle with your weight will be a thing of the past.

Blessings,

Cathy

We pray this book has been a blessing to you. If it has... please don't keep it a secret! Please help others to also be blessed by taking a minute to leave an honest review where this book was purchased.
Thank you.

Guiding Light Publishing

Continue the **journey!**

Lose weight, God's way in our *21-Day Intensive Course* **'The Breakthrough Method'**

21 Daily Insights
and Videos from
Cathy Morenzie

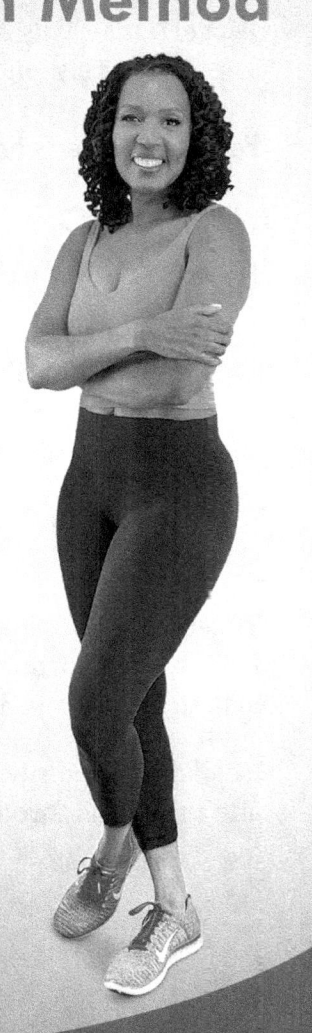

21daysgodsway.com

Weight Loss God's Way Offerings

Weight Loss God's Way (www.weightlossgodsway.com) equips women to rely on God as their strength so they can live in freedom, joy, and peace. At the end of the day, that's what we really want. Let's be honest, if you never achieved that mythical, elusive number on the scale, but were fully able to live a life of freedom, joy, and peace, would that be enough? I know for me the answer is a resounding 'YES!!!'

We provide a multidimensional approach to releasing weight. It encompasses the whole person—spiritual, psychological, mental, nutritional, physical, and even hormonal! We believe that you must address the whole person—body, soul, and spirit.

If you're looking for a program that just tells you what to eat and what exercises to do, this isn't it.

These programs have helped thousands of women break free from all the roadblocks that have been hindering their weight loss success while discovering their identity in Christ.

Weight Loss God's Way offers a variety of free and paid courses and programs throughout the year:

www.weightlossgodsway.com

Weight Loss God's Way Devotional Newsletter

Join the free *Weight Loss God's Way* community and receive regular posts designed to help you align your weight loss with God's Word. You'll also receive a special bonus gift just for joining. To join the newsletter, sign up at:

cathymorenzie.com

Books and Devotionals

You can find all of my weight loss books here:

Christianweightlossbooks.com

Keynote Speaking

Want me to visit your hometown? Need a speaker for your annual conference or special event? My fun and practical approach to *Weight Loss God's Way* will give your group clarity and focus to move toward their weight loss goals. To learn more or to book a speaking engagement, visit:

https://www.cathymorenzie.com/speaking/

Private Coaching

Prefer a more one-on-one approach? I have a few dedicated time slots available to coach you individually to help you fast track your results. To learn more, go to:

https://www.cathymorenzie.com/coach-with-cathy

About The Author

Cathy is a noted personal trainer, author, blogger, and presenter, and has been a leader in the faith/ fitness industry for over a decade. Her impact has influenced hundreds of thousands of people over the years to help them lose weight and develop positive attitudes about their bodies and fitness.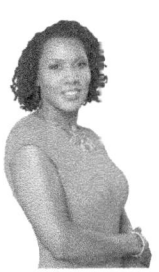

Over the years, she has seen some of the most powerful and faith-filled people struggle with their health and their weight.

Cathy Morenzie herself—a rational, disciplined, faith-filled personal trainer—struggled with her own weight, emotional eating, self-doubt, and low self-esteem. She tried to change just about everything about herself for much of her life, so she knows what it's like to feel stuck. Every insecurity, challenge, and negative emotion that she experienced has equipped her to help other people who face the same struggles—especially women.

With her *Healthy by Design* books and *Weight Loss, God's Way* programs, Cathy has helped thousands to learn to let go of their mental, emotional, and spiritual bonds that have kept them stuck, and instead rely on their Heavenly Father for true release from their fears, doubts, stress, and anxiety. She also teaches people how to eat a sustainable, nutritious diet, and find the motivation to exercise.

Learn more at www.cathymorenzie.com.

Follow Cathy at:

https://www.facebook.com/weightlossgodsway/

youtube.com/@CathyMorenzieWeightLossGodsWay

https://www.pinterest.ca/cathymorenzie

instagram.com/cathy.morenzie

www.ingramcontent.com/pod-product-compliance
Lightning Source LLC
Chambersburg PA
CBHW051006140626
46546CB00016B/960